The Easy Acid Reflux Cookbook

A Cookbook And Lifestyle Guide For Healing GERD And LRP Naturally

Louis Gardner

ISBN: 9781077742536

Limit of Liability

The information in this book is solely for informational purposes, not as a medical instruction to replace the advice of your physician or as a replacement for any treatment prescribed by your physician. The author and publisher do not take responsibility for any possible consequences from any treatment, procedure, exercise, dietary modification, action or application of medication which results from reading or following the information contained in this book.

If you are ill or suspect that you have a medical problem, we strongly encourage you to consult your medical, health, or other competent professional before adopting any of the suggestions in this book or drawing inferences from it.

This book and the author's opinions are solely for informational and educational purposes. The author specifically disclaims all responsibility for any liability, loss, or risk, personal or otherwise which is incurred as a consequence, directly or indirectly, of the use and application of any of the contents of this book.

DEDICATION

To all who desire to live life to the fullest!

TABLE OF CONTENT

INTRODUCTION

WHAT IS ACID REFLUX

Acid reflux is a common digestive condition that characterizes a sensational burning pain in the chest area known as heartburn. It occurs when the acid in the stomach enters into the food pipe.

Generally, most people get confused about the difference between Acid Reflux, Gastro esophageal reflux disease (GERD) and Heartburn.
The word acid reflux, GERD and heartburn are often used without differentiation but these three digestive disorders are different from one another. It's normal to have experience heartburn at some point in life-that burning sensational pain you feel in the chest after a sumptuous meal. While having this pains occasional might not mean anything serious, but when the sensational pain occurs more than once or twice in a week or becomes something that disturbs your sleep, that is sure thing to worry about and might indicate you have gastro esophageal reflux disease (GERD). At this stage, it is advised to visit the doctor.

Acid reflux is a condition or disease that causes you heartburn. It is the major reason you are experiencing that symptoms because stomach acid has escaped into the esophagus. Naturally when food is consumed, it is expected to be transported to the stomach through the esophageal. Lower esophageal sphincter (LES) is a collection of muscles that gives way for the fluid or food to pass through the stomach and obstruct any content from the stomach from entering the esophagus.

Reflux is a declining condition of the lower esophageal sphincter (LES) and whenever you experience Acid reflux does not translate to a chronic condition. Whenever there is a malfunctioning in the function of the LES, what you are experiencing is a reflux. So, whether you have reflux once a month or once a year, the bottom line is you are still regarded to have acid reflux.

Heartburn is one of the many symptom of acid reflux and gastro-esophageal reflux disease (GERD) and the most common of the all. Heartburn is never a disease or condition. It is a situation where you have a burning pain in the lower chest as results of the stomach contents finding a way into the esophagus.

GERD is a chronic digestive condition affecting the lower esophageal sphincter (LES) that cause the continuous inflow of stomach acid into the esophagus. Most patient are diagnosed with GERD if they frequently experience heartburn or other reflux symptoms, like two times or more in a week. It may not be necessary to treat Acid reflux, but treating GERD is important.

Sadly more than 100 million Americans have acid reflux without realizing they have this condition

CAUSES OF ACID REFLUX

Why do we have so many people with acid reflux condition? Acid reflux condition may be as a result of many reasons.

Let's see some of common causes of acid reflux disease. One major reason is the increased rate of acid in most of the foods we eat, especially canned or bottled foods

In this present era, some of the so called canned or bottled foods contain as much acid as that of the stomach itself.

Stomach abnormalities: This is another reason for acid reflux disease known as hiatal hernia. Hiatal hernia occurs as a result of the higher section of the stomach and lower esophageal sphincter (LES) moved above the diaphragm. These abnormalities can happen in persons of any age.

Diaphragm: This is the muscle enclosure that divides the stomach and the chest. A proper functional diaphragm usually helps prevent acid from springing up into the esophagus. But hiatal hernia condition will make it easy for acid to rise into your esophagus.

Smoking. Smoking may be a contributing factor to acid reflux condition through any of the following:

Reducing salivation, which neutralizes the effect of acid
Reducing LES muscle function
Increasing acid secretion
Impairing muscle reflexes in the throat
Damaging mucus membranes

Pregnancy: Most pregnant women encounter acid reflux, especially during their first pregnancy period. This occurs by rising levels of hormones integrating with pressure from the developing fetus. Worst during the third trimester, the symptoms usually almost vanished after delivery.

Other Common Causes Of Acid Reflux Disease Include:

Obesity or overweight
Eating a sumptuous meal and lying down on your back after meal
Going to bed immediately after eating or lying down immediately after a meal
Taking some certain blood pressure medications or muscle relaxers

Some of the common Symptoms of Acid Reflux Disease
Heartburn: It's a condition where you have a burning pain in the lower chest as a result of the stomach contents finding a way into the esophagus.
Regurgitation:
Regurgitation is the forcibly ejection of food from the stomach or esophagus without nausea.
Other symptoms of acid reflux disease include:
Chronic sore throat
Dry cough
Wheezing
Hoarseness
Weight loss
Nausea
Hiccups that don't let up
Dysphagia -- a physical feeling of food being stuck in your throat
Burping
Bloody vomiting or Bloody or black stools
Bloating

Chest pain

List Of Some Of The Common Foods That Trigger Acid Reflux Symptoms:

Citrus fruits, such as lemons or oranges
Coffee or tea (decaffeinated or regular)
Chocolate
Carbonated beverages
Alcohol
Fried orFatty foods
Foods containing tomato, such as pizza, salsa, or spaghetti sauce
Garlic and onions
Mint
Spicy foods
Excessive alcohol drinking can also heighten the risk of esophageal cancer. Regular drinkers have a greater risk than occasional drinkers. When excessive drinking is mixed with smoking, the risk becomes greater than using either tobacco or alcohol alone.

Ways To Prevention Heartburn

Limit the amount of food you eat to smaller Servings.

Be sensitive to food that triggers your heartburn. There is a long list of heartburn triggering by researchers, study list to know what triggers your heartburn.

These includes spicy foods, alcohol, carbonated beverages, citrus fruits and juices, coffee and caffeine, tomato sauce chocolate, mint, and fatty foods.

Fatty foods takes longer time leaving the stomach; therefore, reduce the overall amount of fatty food consumption by cutting down the amount of fatty meats, oils , butter, margarine, gravy, salad dressings, and full-fat dairy/milk products like whole milk, cheese and sour cream.

Rely on Gravity
A good way to suppress nighttime reflux is by making use of gravity, you can use a wedge-shaped pillow to lift up your upper body at night. You can also add few inches to the head of your bed to elevate and help keep stomach contents from rising.

Try to always remain upright after a meal. You can take a brief walk after a big meal without overdoing it.
Avoid wearing clothes that is tight in the abdominal area.
Chewing Gum after an attack or a meal helps to relieve heartburn but avoid mint-flavored gums.

Get Healthy
Researchers have confirmed that people who smoke are prone to heartburn. To avoid GERD, quit smoking to reduce the risk of acid reflux.

There is a direct relationship between being overweight and heartburn. That little extra pound can increase the pressure on the stomach and the esophagus. So take care of yourself and try shedding those extra pounds.

Maintain an upright posture while eating and about 45-60 minutes afterward, avoid bending over or reaching below your waist after meals to do things like loading the dishwasher, tying your shoes, or picking up items from the ground.

DIETARY LIFESTYLE GUIDELINES FOR THE TREATMENT OF GERD

The following list of food can help you choose what to eat to reduce stomach reflux. Tolerances may differ from person to persons.

Milk and milk products
These foods are generally regarded safe: Reduced- Fat, free-fat or low-fat, yogurt, reduced- Fat, low-fat, and free-fat milk, low-fat cottage cheese, soy milk.

Possible trigger foods: whole milk fat (4%) cottage cheese, whole milk fat yogurt, chocolate drinks or shakes, milkshakes, whole milk, chocolate milk, cereals and full-fat cheese.

Breads
These foods are generally regarded safe: Plain bread (with whole grain flour or without whole grain flour), corntortillas, waffles, crackers, rolls, low-fat ingredients muffins, pancakes, bagels, cereals.

Possible trigger foods: Breads with cereals made with high-fat ingredients like biscuits, pizza, sweet rolls, doughnuts, granola, muffins, and croissants.

Desserts
These foods are generally regarded safe: Low-fat cookies, fruit ice, reduced-fat ice cream, fat-free pudding sponge cake, gelatin, sherbet, fruit-based desserts, custard or pudding prepared with 1% or 2% low-fat milk, Angel food cake.

Possible trigger foods: ice cream, cakes and cookies, all other pies, desserts with chocolate frosting, pastries, whole milk pudding.

Fats
These foods are generally regarded safe: Cream cheese and sour cream, fat-free or non-fat dressing, mayo, powdered or liquid creamer, reduced- fat or Low-fat products, margarine or butter (But not more than 8 teaspoon per day.)

Possible trigger foods: Cream cheeses, guacamole, bacon, olives, meat drippings, margarine, butter, regular sour cream, vegetable oils, gravies, heavy cream, nut butters, vegetable oils (Limit to less than 4 tsp per day.)

Fruits
These foods are generally regarded safe: canned, frozen, and fresh, fruits as tolerated, all juices (with the exception of those listed as trigger foods)
Possible trigger foods: pineapple, lemon, Orange lime, grapefruit, tangerine.

Meats and meat substitutes

These foods are generally regarded safe: Poultry (without skin),shellfish, well-cooked lean meat, low-fat hot dogs, fresh or water-packed fish, low-fat luncheon cheeses and meats, eggs, tofu, lean pork, peas and dried beans (includes fat-free refried beans)

Possible trigger foods: Fried versions of Fish, meat, eggs or poultry; regular luncheon meats, sausages, refried beans, hot dogs, nuts.

Potatoes and potato substitutes

These foods are generally regarded safe: Boiled, baked, and mashed without added fat, low-fat cream sauce pasta, plain pasta, rice.

Possible trigger foods: Risotto, potato chips, french-fried potatoes, tomato-based sauces and pastas served with cream sauces.

Soups

Foods that are generally considered safe: Fat-free or low-fat milk, fat-free broths, soups prepared with vegetables lean meat (without tomatoes).

Possible trigger foods: Tomato-based soups and Regular cream.

Sweets

These foods are generally regarded safe: Maple syrup, marshmallows, hard candy, jam, honey, molasses, jelly, sugar

Possible trigger foods: peppermint, cream-filled candies, chocolate, nuts, spearmint, coconut.

Vegetables
These foods are generally regarded safe: frozen, canned and plain fresh vegetables made without added fat.

Possible trigger foods: Onions creamed or fried vegetables, vegetable juices, tomatoes and tomato products.
Miscellaneous
These foods are generally regarded safe: non-mint tea, decaffeinated tea, pepper, herbs and spices and (as tolerated), decaffeinated coffee, sage, oregano, salt.

Possible trigger foods: Jalapeno and chili peppers, herbs and Spices in tomato-based sauces, carbonated beverages, vinegar, alcoholic beverages, mint-flavored or caffeinated teas or coffee.

BREAKFAST RECIPES

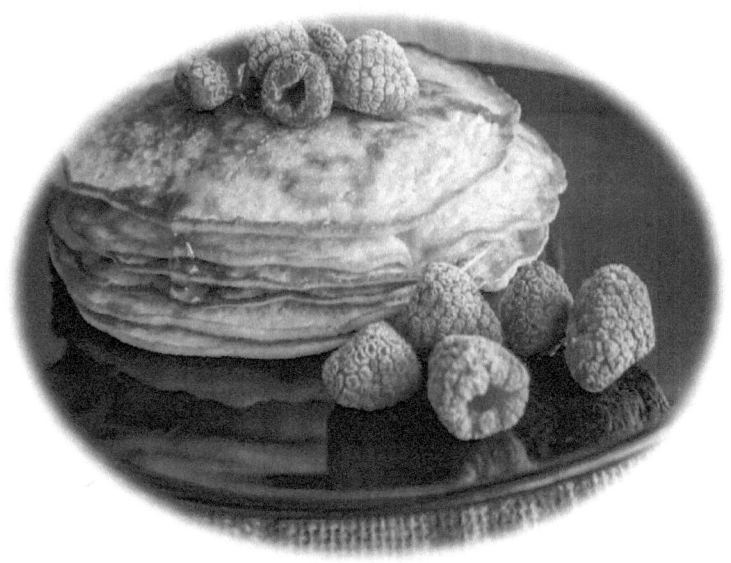

Heartburn-Friendly Oatmeal

Prep time: 5 minutes
Cook time: 5 minutes
Servings: 1

INGREDIENTS

2 Cup of Almond Milk
1 1/4 Cup of Quick Oats
2 tablespoon of Flax Seeds Crushed
2 teaspoon of ground cinnamon
2 teaspoon of Vanilla Extract
2 Cup of Water
1/2 Cup of Fresh Blueberries
2 teaspoon of Walnuts Chopped
1 teaspoon of Manuka Honey

INSTRUCTIONS

1. Add water with the oats into a pan over medium high heat and bring to boil, stirring frequently. Stir in the cinnamon, vanilla extract and flax seeds; keep cooking 2 to 3 minutes more until water is no more and oats is tender.
2. Add the blueberries and almond milk and stir into the oatmeal.
Transfer into a bowl and stir in the honey. Top with walnuts.

Nutrition information per servings:
Calories: 782 kcal
Carbohydrates: 98 g
Fat: 22gg
Protein: 24g
Sodium: 190 mg

Breakfast Smoothie

Prep time: 5 minutes

Cook time: 5 minutes

Servings: 2

INGREDIENTS

1/2 Cup of ice

1 tablespoon of Honey

1/2 teaspoon of ginger Peeled and grated

1 Cup of Unsweetened Yogurt

2 Small ripe Bananas, peel

2 Cups of Low-fat milk

INSTRUCTIONS

1. Roughly chop the bananas and place in a blender. Add milk, ice, ginger and yogurt.

Blend ingredients together till smooth.

2. Pour in 1 tablespoon honey and blend once more for few seconds.

Place in the refrigerator to chill the smoothie.

Nutrition information per servings:

Calories: 333 kcal

Carbohydrates: 57 g

Fat: 2g

Protein: 14g

Sodium: 169 mg

Meseli Breakfast

Prep time: 5 minutes
Cook time: 5 minutes
Servings: 2

INGREDIENTS

1/4 cup of dried chopped apricots
1/4 (20 ounces) cup of raisins
1 1/4 cup of natural yogurt
1/2 santrail farms lemon
2 1/4 cup of oats
2 eating resedene farm apples
2 cups of almond milk
1/4 cup of flaked almond
1/2 cup of orange juice
Fresh berries to serve

INSTRUCTIONS

1. Mix together in a bowl the grated apple, oats, apricot, almonds and raisin
2. Mix in orange, lemon and milk mix well and place in the refrigerator overnight

Spread the yogurt on it and serve.

Nutrition information per servings:
Calories: 462 kcal
Carbohydrates: 109 g
Fat: 1.5g
Protein: 4.5g

Asparagus AndCarrots, Green Bean Salad

Prep time: 10 minutes

Cook time: 8 minutes

Servings: 12

INGREDIENTS

3 tablespoons of olive oil

4 teaspoons of balsamic vinegar

2 teaspoons of Dijon mustard

3 hard-boiled eggs, cut into quarters

3 to 4 turkey bacon slices, cooked and crumbled

2 tablespoons of shredded carrots

1 lbs of French beans, stems removed

1 lbs of fresh asparagus

Dash of salt and pepper

INSTRUCTIONS

1. Pour water into a large pot and bring to a boil.Add fresh asparagus and beans, bring to a boil, then reduce heat and simmer until tender, about 4 minutes. (Do not overcook)

2. Drain the asparagus and beans from the pot, rinse using cold water. Store the asparagus and beans in the fridge to chill.

3. Whisk olive oil, Dijon mustard, balsamic vinegar and salt and pepper to taste for the vinaigrette.

4. Chop the cooled asparagus and beans, place in a salad bowl, sprinkle with bacon and carrots. Drizzle salad with vinaigrette and place eggs slices on top.

Nutrition information per servings:

Calories: 211 kcal

Carbohydrates: g

Fat: 1g;

Protein: g

Sodium 295 mg

Black Bean Burger

Prep time: 10 minutes

Cook time: 10 minutes

Servings: 6

INGREDIENTS

6 whole wheat buns

Iceberg lettuce

Pineapple slices, Divided

1/4 cup of vegetable oil

1/2 cup of baked tortilla chips, crushed

1/4 teaspoon of salt

1/4 teaspoon of pepper

1/2 teaspoon of ground coriander

1 teaspoons of ground cumin

2 tablespoons of minced cilantro

2 tablespoon of Flour

1/3 cup of chopped green pepper

2 eggs

2-15 oz cans of black beans, drained

INSTRUCTIONS

1. Place 3 layers of paper towels over a rimmed baking sheet and place the drained beans over. Allow to sit for about 20 minutes.

2. Mash eggs with drained beans, flour, crushed tortilla chips and seasonings in a large bowl.

3. Shape mixture evenly into six patties and chill in the refrigerator for an hour.

4. In a nonstick skillet, heat one tablespoon of vegetable oil. Place three burgers carefully into the pan and cook for 5 minutes. Turnover and cook the other side for 3 to 4 minutes

more or until crisp. Remove burgers from the skillet and keep warm. Repeat.

5. Serve burgers on whole wheat buns along GERD friendly condiments, add pineapple to the top.

Nutrition information per servings:
Calories: 360 kcal
 Carbohydrates: g;
Fat: 1g;
Protein: g
Sodium 697 mg

Mashed Banana Walnut Muffins

Prep time: 15 minutes
Cook time: 17-20 minutes
Servings: 18 muffins

INGREDIENTS

1/2 cup of grated dried unsweetened coconut

1/2 cup chopped walnuts

1 teaspoon of vanilla extract

3 very ripe bananas, mashed with a fork

2 eggs

1/3 cup of coconut oil

3/4 cup of sugar

1 1/2 teaspoon of baking powder

1 teaspoon of salt

2 cup of whole wheat flour

INSTRUCTIONS

1. Heat up your oven to 375 F. Line muffin tin with cupcake liners or grease the muffin tin.

2. Combine the dry ingredients together in a bowl.

3. Beat the eggs in another bowl and mix with coconut oil plus mashed bananas.
4. Add banana/egg mixture into the dry mix and stir until finely combined.
5. Add in the walnuts, vanilla and coconut and gently stir.
6. Scoop mixture into muffin tins, 2/3 full.
7. Place in the oven and bake for 17-20 minutes until set. It is set when you insert a toothpick into the middle and it comes out clean.
8. Let muffins stand in the pan, out of the oven for about 5 minutes before transferring onto a cooling rack.

You can consume sugar in small measure without added trigger ingredients. This will not affect your acid reflux.Maple syrup, jams, and pure honeys will not trigger any symptoms. Avoid Sugar combined with triggering ingredients or sugar found in triggering foods.

Nutrition information per servings:
Calories: 218 kcal
 Carbohydrates: 23g
Fat: 9g
Protein: 3g
Sodium 139 mg

Coated Chicken cutlets Andmushrooms

Prep time: 7 minutes
Cook time: 11 minutes
Servings: 4

INGREDIENTS

1/3 cup of low sodium chicken broth or white wine
2 cups of mushrooms, sliced
3 tbsp of butter
2 tbsp of olive oil
1/3 cup of whole wheat flour
1 lbs of skinless, boneless chicken cutlets
Salt and pepper to taste

INSTRUCTIONS

1. Season chicken cutlets with pepper and salt.
2. Pour the whole wheat flour into a bowl; dip the chicken into the bowl to lightly coat in flour.
3. Heat the olive oil over medium high heat in a large skillet. Brown the chicken on both sides in the skillet. (3-4 minutes per side). Set aside.
4. Reduce to medium heat. Add in butter with slices of mushrooms and sauté about 5 minute until mushrooms are soft.
5. Add low sodium chicken broth or white wine and deglaze the pan.
6. Place browned chicken into the skillet and cook about 2 minutes until sauce is thickened. Serve and enjoy!

Nutrition information per servings:
Calories: 289 kcal
Carbohydrates: 9g
Fat: 18g
Protein: 26g
Sodium 329 mg

Asparagus Turkey Bacon Quiche

Prep time: 15 minutes

Cook time: 45 minutes

Servings: 4

INGREDIENTS

½ Cup of Swiss cheese

1 ½ Cup of low- fat plain yogurt or nonfat (You can also use Greek yogurt but flavor may be more tart)

3 eggs (or 2 eggs and 2 egg whites/ 1 egg and 3 egg whites)

2 tablespoons of green onion or chives

6 strips of turkey bacon, cooked crispy and chopped

½ lbs of asparagus, cut into ¼ inch pieces

1 unbaked, 9-inch piecrust

¼ Cup of Parmesan cheese

1/8 teaspoon of nutmeg

½ teaspoon of salt

INSTRUCTIONS

1. Heat up your oven to 450 degrees, cover the piecrust with foil and place in the oven Bake for five minutes, discard foil and bake for 5 more minutes.

2. Steam the asparagus about 4-5 minutes or until tender, crisp and bright green.

3. Meanwhile, beat together the eggs in a mixing bowl and gradually add in the yogurt, half cup at a time.

4. Stir in the chives, nutmeg and salt.

5. Gradually add cheeses, but reserve small to sprinkle over the quiche.

6. Add cooked bacon to the egg mixture.

7. Once the asparagus has been steamed and piecrust is finished baking, spread the asparagus onto the base of the piecrust.

8. Gently add yogurt/egg mixture on the top the asparagus

9. Sprinkle top of the quiche with the reserved cheese.

10. Place the quiche in the oven and bake for 10 minutes at 400F, then reduce oven heat to 350F and keep baking for 25-30 minutes or until a knife inserted into the quiche comes out clean.

11. Allow to stand for 15-20 minutes before serving or else the quiche will fall apart.

Nutrition information per servings:

Calories: 200 kcal;

Carbohydrates: 2g;

Fat: 11g;

Protein: 10g;

Sodium 335 mg;

Friendly Whole Wheat Banana Walnut Scones

Prep time: 10 minutes

Cook time: 15-20 minutes

Servings: 4

INGREDIENTS

1/4 cup of walnut pieces

1 mashed banana

2/3 cup of plain non-fat yogurt

1/2 cup of smart balance

1/2 teaspoon of baking soda

1 teaspoon of baking powder

2 tablespoons of ground flax seeds

¼ cup of brown sugar

1 1/4cup of whole wheat flour

1 1/4 cup of oatmeal

1/4 cup of mini chocolate chips (Optional)

INSTRUCTIONS

1. Whisk the flour, baking powder, oatmeal, sugar, flax seeds and soda together in a bowl.

2. Add in the Smart Balance and blend with a fork or pastry blender until mixture resemble coarse crumbs.

3. Add in mashed banana and yogurt and stir until mixture is well incorporated. Stir in chocolate chips with walnuts.

4. Scoop the mixture with an ice cream scoop, place on a parchment paper or wax paper lined cookie sheet. Alternatively, you can also make the mixture into a big circle and use a knife to cut into 8 scones like a pizza.

5. To prevent the bottoms from burning, Stack 2 cookies sheets, then bake for 15-20 minutes at 400 degrees.

Nutrition information per servings:
Calories: 196 kcal
Carbohydrates: 4g
Fat: 7g
Protein: 6g
Sodium 100 mg

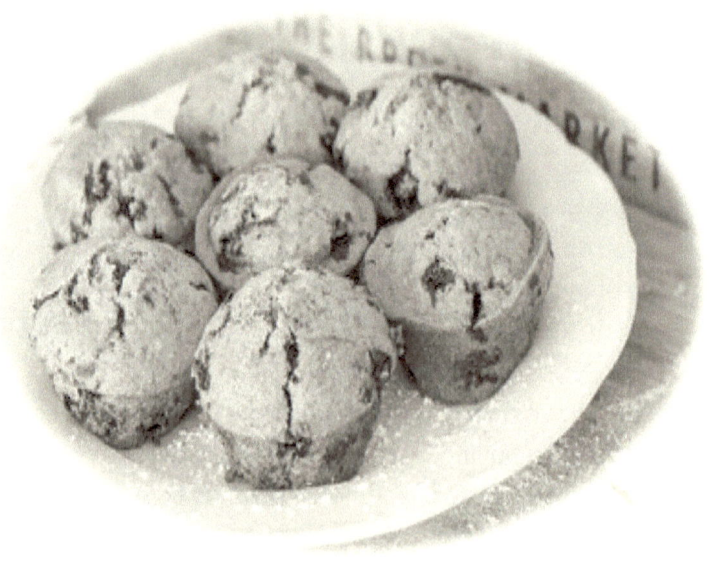

Easy Poached Salmon

Prep time: 5 minutes
Cook time: 15 minutes
Servings: 4

INGREDIENTS

1 tsp of olive oil
4 half-slice fresh lemon
4 sprigs fresh rosemary
4 (4 ounces each) salmon filets

INSTRUCTIONS

1. Lay each of the salmon filet on a large sheet of aluminum foil, skin-side down.
2. Place rosemary and lemon on the salmon and drizzle with ¼ teaspoon of olive oil. Season with salt to taste.
3. Wrap foil around each filet and transfer onto a baking pan, place in the oven and bake for 10-15 minutes at 350°F.
4. Once done, remove from oven and remove the foil, discard the rosemary and lemon (You don't need to squeeze the lemon over the filet).
5. Serve with your favorite steamed greens and rice.

Nutrition information per servings:
Calories: 514 kcal
Carbohydrates: 82g
Fat: 4g
Protein: 38g

Sweet Potato and Green Bean

Prep time: 10 minutes

Cook time: 15-20 minutes

Servings: 6

INGREDIENTS

3 cups of baby arugula or watercress

1 tsp of sesame seeds, toasted

2 tbsp of soy sauce

2 bay leaves

Pineapple juice

1/4 tsp of ground cumin

Maple syrup, as desired

1 lemon Zest from (washed, to yield about 2 tsp)

2 tbsp of olive oil

1 pounds of sweet potatoes, peeled and cut into 1-inch cubes

1 pounds of green beans, remove both ends and cut into about 2 inches long pieces

INSTRUCTIONS

1. Cook the green beans in salted boiling water until al dente. Remove immediately and place in ice-cold water.This will prevent the beans from losing the bright green color.Drain.

2. In a small saucepan, place the cumin, pineapple juice with bay leaves. Simmer on low heat until reduced by half. Pour into a bowl.

3. Mix the soy sauce and maple syrup with the pineapple juice mixture in a bowl.

4. Heat olive oil in a skillet on high heat, add potatoes and cook for few minutes until golden brown.

5. In a bowl, place the sweet potatoes and add in lemon zest, green beans and pineapple mixture. Toss together until well mixed.

6. Add the baby arugula into a plate and add the vegetables over top with a sprinkle of toasted sesame seeds. Serve immediately at room temperature.

Notes: Allow potatoes to cool a bit before adding the baby arugula or watercress, else it will wilt.

Nutrition information per servings:
Calories: 253 kcal
Carbohydrates: 39g
Fat: 10g
Protein: 3g

Quick Omelet

Prep time: 5 minutes
Cook time: 5 minutes
Servings: 1
INGREDIENTS
1/2 cup of filling (meat, vegetable, seafood)
1 tbsp of unsalted margarine
2 tbsp of water
2 eggs
INSTRUCTIONS
1. In a bowl, whisk together water and eggs until fluffy.
2. Heat margarine in a fry pan until hot.
3. Add in the egg mixture into the pan and carefully shift the cooked edges to the center and allow the uncooked side flow to the hot pan's surface. Move pan as necessary until the egg is set.

4. If desired, fill the omelet with 1/2 cup meat, vegetable, seafood. Push filling towards your left side.
5. Fold omelet in half with the pancake turner and invert onto a plate.

Nutrition information per servings:
Calories: 257 kcal
Carbohydrates: 20g
Fat: g
Protein: 15g
Sodium 384 mg

Blueberry Pancakes

Prep time: 10 minutes

Cook time: 30 minutes

Servings: 6 (12 pancakes)

INGREDIENTS

1 cup of canned or frozen blueberries, rinsed

2 slightly beaten eggs

2 tbsp of no-salt margarine, melted

1 cup of buttermilk

3 tbsp of brown sugar

2 tsp of baking powder

1 1/2 cups of sifted plain all-purpose flour

INSTRUCTIONS

1. Sift baking powder, flour and sugar together in a mixing bowl.

2. Make a round hole in the middle and pour in the rest ingredients.

Start stirring from the middle and gently stir in the dry ingredients until a smooth batter is formed.

3. Lightly grease a heavy 12-inch griddle or skillet. Heat up the skillet and spoon 1/3 measuring cup of batter in the hot skillet and cook until browned underside, flip and cook the other side.

Nutrition information per servings:

Calories: 223 kcal

Carbohydrates: 35g

Fat: g

Protein: 7g

Sodium 196 mg

Rice Salmon cucumber Salad

Prep Time: 10 minutes
Cook Time: 15 to 20 minutes
Servings: 4

INGREDIENTS

½ cup of salmon, low sodium, drained
1 cooked egg, chopped
½ cup of celery, chopped
½ teaspoon of celery seed
1 teaspoon of horseradish
½ cup of sliced cucumber
1 tablespoon of finely chopped onion
¼ teaspoon of pepper
¼ cup of French dressing
½ cup of rice, uncooked

INSTRUCTIONS

1. Pour two cups of water and rice in a saucepan. Cover with the lid and bring to a boil. Reduce heat to low and simmer, about 15 to 20 minutes until rice is cooked.
2. Transfer rice to a bowl, cover and let sit for 15 minutes.
3. Add the French dressing and allow cooling, then add the rest ingredients.

Allow to chill in the refrigerator for up to an hour.

Nutrition information per servings:
Calories: 236 kcal
Carbohydrate 22g
Fat: g
Protein 8g
Sodium 145 mg

Cornmeal Blueberry Pancakes

Prep time: 10 minutes

Cook time: 30 minutes

Servings: 2 pancakes

INGREDIENTS

1 teaspoon of pure vanilla extract

1/4 cup of egg substitute

2/3 cup of non-fat buttermilk

1/4 teaspoon of salt

1 teaspoon of baking powder

2 teaspoons of Splenda or stevia

1/4 cup of whole wheat flour

1/2 cup of blue cornmeal

2 teaspoons of unsalted butter (per serving)

2 tablespoons of fresh blueberries (per serving)

1 tablespoon of pure maple syrup

INSTRUCTIONS

1. Sift the whole wheat flour, baking powder, blue cornmeal, salt and splenda   in a mixing bowl. Add the vanilla extract, egg substitute and buttermilk and whisk until mixture is smooth. Let stand for two minutes, stir once and leave for another minute before adding to the hot skillet.

2. Meanwhile, heat a non-stick skillet/griddle over high-medium heat. Once hot, reduce to medium heat and add the batter to the skillet/griddle (about 1/4 cups each).

3. Once it is one minute into the cooking, spread one tbsp. of blueberries on top each pancakes.

4. Cook for 1 to 2 minutes until the surface form bubbles and burst. Flip and cook the other side for 30 seconds to 1 minutes until golden brown.

5. Transfer onto a plate and top 1 tsp of unsalted butter on each pancake and serve one tbsp. pure maple syrup on 2 pancakes.

Note: Those that are lactose intolerant and sensitive to gluten may avoid this recipe.

Nutrition information per servings:
Calories: 363 kcal
Carbohydrates: 56g
Fat: 8g
Protein: 13g
Sodium 322 mg

Shredded Sweet Potato Hash Browns

Prep time: 5 minutes
Cook time: 30 minutes
Servings: 1 cup

INGREDIENTS

2 teaspoon of unsalted butter
Fresh ground black pepper (to taste)
1 teaspoon of dried sage
1/8 teaspoon ofsalt
8 oz of sweet potatoes

INSTRUCTIONS

1. Shred the potatoes and transfer into a strainer. Force any excess water out of the potatoes using the back of a rubber spatula.
2. Lay two paper towel on each other and place the potatoes to pat dry as you can.
3. In a bowl, place the potatoes, add pepper, sage and salt and toss together until well blended.

4. Heat the unsalted butter on a large skillet/griddle over medium high heat. Once melted, add in the potatoes.
5. Toss for about five minutes, then separate into 2 piles. Press each piles down to flatten.
6. Reduce to medium heat and cook potatoes slowly about 5 minutes without burning. Turn and cook for 3 to 5 minutes on the other side. Serve.

Nutrition information per servings:
Calories: 169 kcal
Carbohydrates: 27g
Fat: 4g
Protein: 2g
Sodium 156 mg

Roasted Yams With Tortilla

Prep time:10 minutes

Cook time: 45 minutes

Servings: 4

INGREDIENTS

1 oz of grated Parmigiano-Reggiano

Fresh ground black pepper (to taste)

1/4 teaspoon of paprika

1/8 teaspoon of salt

2 teaspoons of fresh minced oregano

1/4 cup of fresh cilantro (chopped coarsely)

1 tablespoon of water

4 large eggs

1 diced mediumred onion

1 minced clove garlic

2 teaspoon of extra virgin olive oil

8 oz of yams

INSTRUCTIONS

1. Heat up your oven to 325°F.

2. Roast yam for 30 minutes in the oven; once soft, open oven and transfer the yam to a bowl. Allow to cool slightly then mash with a fork.

3. In a non-stick skillet (8 inch), heat the olive oil over medium heat and place the garlic. Allow to cook about a minute then pour in the onions. Cook stirring constantly until onions are soft and golden brown.

4. Add the onions with the mashed yams and fold together.

5. In a bowl, whisk the water, eggs, oregano, cilantro, paprika, pepper and salt together.

6. Pour egg/oregano mixture into the pan and fold with the yam/onion mixture.

7. Place in the preheated oven and cook until the center is set, about 20 minutes. To serve, top with the grated cheese.

Nutrition information per servings:
Calories: 388 kcal
Carbohydrates: 11g
Fat: 10g
Protein: 21g
Sodium 525 mg

Berry's French Toast

Prep time: 5 minutes
Cook time: 30 minutes
Servings: 2 slices

INGREDIENTS

4 1 oz of slices sourdough bread
1/8 teaspoon ofsalt
1/2 teaspoon ofpure vanilla extract
1/4 teaspoon ofground nutmeg
6 tablespoons of 2% milk
2 teaspoons of Splenda or stevia
6 tablespoons of egg substitute
 1 tablespoon of pure maple syrup (per serving)
2 teaspoons of unsalted butter (per serving)

INSTRUCTIONS

1. In a large mixing bowl, whisk together the milk, egg substitute, vanilla, ground nutmeg, Splenda and salt until finely blended.

2. Heat a skillet over medium-high heat, once hot, lower heat to medium. Dip four bread slices into the batter. Carefully coat the bread slices in the batter until coated well and soaked slightly.
3. Place the coated bread slices on the skillet and cook for 3 to 4 minutes. Flip over and cook the other side. Cook, turning periodically until golden brown on both sides. You may need to reduce heat slightly, depending on your skillet or stove.
4. Remove from the skillet and top each with 1 tsp butter and serve one tbsp pure maple syrup on 2 French toast slices.

Note: Those that are lactose intolerant and sensitive to gluten may wish to avoid this recipe

Nutrition information per servings:
Calories: 346 kcal
Carbohydrates: 53g
Fat: 7g
Protein: 15g

French Toast with Apple

Prep time: 5 minutes

Cook time: 10 minutes

Servings: 2

INGREDIENTS

¾ (175 mL) cup of apple sauce

½ (125 mL) cup of milk

4 slices white bread

2 lightly beaten eggs

INSTRUCTIONS

1. Beat together the milk and eggs in a bowl, add apple sauce.

2. Heat a nonstick pan on medium high heat; melt a dot of olive oil in the pan.

3. Take each bread slice and soak in mixture.

4. Cook soaked bread slices in the pan until browned underside, then flip and cook the other side. Serve and top with syrup.

Nutrition information per servings:

Calories: 352 kcal

Carbohydrates: 60g

Fat: g

Protein: 12g

Sodium 462mg

Easy Quinoa And Qats Granola

Prep time: 10 minutes

Cook time: 75 minutes

Servings: 6

INGREDIENTS

1/4 cup of dried cranberries

1/4 cup of raisins

2 tablespoons of pure maple syrup

1/8 teaspoon of salt

1/2 teaspoon of ground nutmeg

1/2 teaspoon of ground cinnamon

1/2 cup of unsweetened applesauce

1/4 cup of chopped walnuts

1/4 cup of sliced almonds

2/3 cup of quinoa

1 1/3 cups of steel cut oats

3 quarts of water

INSTRUCTIONS

1. Heat up your oven to 300°F.

1. Boil water over high heat in a large sauce pan, then add the quinoa and oats to the boiling water. Lower heat and simmer for 12 minutes. Drain water from quinoa and oats and rinse with cold water.

2. Arrange the drained quinoa and oats in a large bowl, add the walnuts, almonds, maple syrup, cinnamon, applesauce, nutmeg, salt, cranberries and raisins. Mix until nicely blended.

3. Line a large cookie sheet with aluminum foil and Spread the mixture flat.

4. Transfer to the oven and bake about 45 minutes. Stirring with a fork every 10 minutes. Remove and allow to cool completely before storing.

Nutrition information per servings:

Calories: 239 kcal

Carbohydrates: 35g

Fat: 7g

Protein: 8g

Orange French Toast breakfast

Prep time: 7 minutes

Cook time: 30 minutes

Servings: 2 slices

INGREDIENTS

1/2 teaspoon of Grand Marnier

2 tablespoons of honey

2 tsp of unsalted butter (per serving)

4 slices of sourdough bread

1/4 teaspoon of grated orange peel

1/4 cup of orange juice

1/4 teaspoon ofpure vanilla extract

1 tablespoon of 2% milk

1 tablespoon of Splenda or stevia

2 teaspoons of Grand Marnier orange liqueur

3 ounces of egg substitute

INSTRUCTIONS

1. In a large mixing bowl, whisk together the milk, Grand Mariner, egg substitute, vanilla, orange peel, Splenda and orange juice until finely blended.

2. Heat a skillet over medium-high heat. Once hot, lower heat to medium, and dip four bread slices into the batter. Carefully coat the bread slices in the batter until coated well and soaked slightly.

3. Place the coated bread slices on the skillet and cook for 3 to 4 minutes. Flip overand cook the other side. Cook, turning once periodically until golden brown on both sides. You may need to reduce heat slightly, depending on your skillet or stove.

4. Remove from the skillet and top each with 1 tsp Take Control Light spread and serve 1 tbsp orange honey on 2 French toast slices.

Nutrition information per servings:
Calories: 342 kcal
Carbohydrates: 57g
Fat: 6g
Protein: 11g
Sodium 523mg

BEEF AND MEAT RECIPES

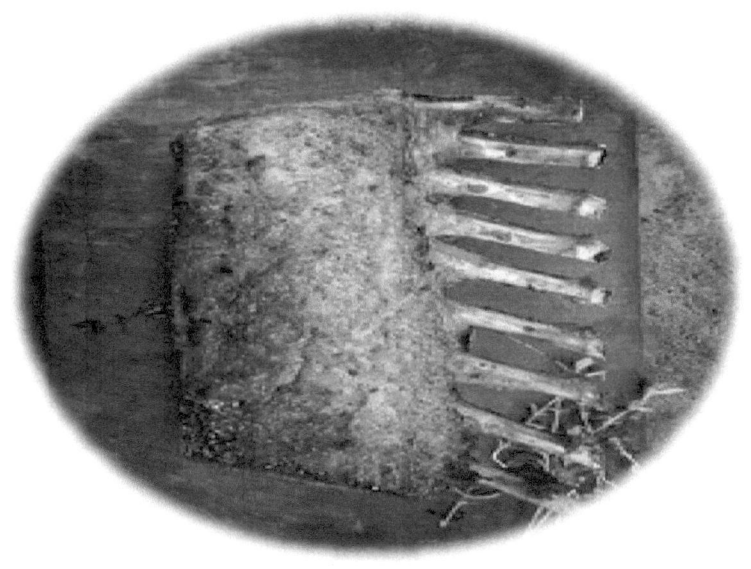

Five Spice Asian Steak

Prep time: 10minutes

Cook time: 30 minutes

Servings: 2

INGREDIENTS

1 teaspoons of unsalted butter

4 tablespoons of gluten-free beer

8 oz of flank steak

Fresh ground black pepper (to taste)

1/2 teaspoons of five spice powder

3 teaspoons of low sodium soy sauce or gluten-free tamari sauce

1 teaspoons of toasted sesame oil

4 teaspoons of fresh minced ginger

4 cloves of roasted garlic

INSTRUCTIONS

1. Place the soy sauce, ginger, sesame oil, five spice and garlic powder in a blender and pulse until smooth.

2. Heat up your oven to 400°Degrees F and place a skillet.

3. Sprinkle pepper on the steak and place into the hot pan.

4. Pour sauce into the skillet, turning the steak until coated on both sides.

5. Cook for eight minutes, flip and cook for 7-9 extra minutes for medium rare.

6. Remove the skillet and transfer the steak onto a cutting board.

7. Pour the beer into the skillet and stir well to deglaze the skillet. Add in butter and whisk to smoothen. Serve the steak with the sauce with Mashed Yams or Plain Mashed Potatoes and Pan Grilled Broccoli.

Nutrition information per servings:
Calories: 259 kcal
Carbohydrates: 8g
Fat: 12g
Protein: 25g
Sodium 330mg

Fancy Meatballs

Prep time: 5 minutes
Cook time: 60 minutes
Servings: 24 meatballs

INGREDIENTS

Spray olive oil
1/8 teaspoon of fresh ground black pepper
1/2 teaspoon of salt
1 teaspoon of dried thyme
1 teaspoon of dried rosemary
1 teaspoon of dried basil
1 teaspoon of dried oregano
2 oz of fresh bread crumbs
1 pounds of extra lean beef (7% fat)

INSTRUCTIONS

1. Heat up your oven to 400°Degrees F and place a skillet.
2. Mix together the bread crumbs, ground beef, rosemary, oregano, thyme, basil, pepper and salt until well mixed.
3. Form mixture with your palms into 24 small balls.
4. Lightly spritz the hot pan with olive oil. Add the meatballs into the pan and place in the oven. Cook until meatballs are firm to touch, about 12 – 15 minutes

Nutrition information per servings:

Calories: 219 kcal

Carbohydrates: 10g

Fat: 11g

Protein: 26g

Sodium 470mg

Herb Seasoned Rib Eye Steak

Prep time: 10 minutes

Cook time: 30 minutes

Servings: 4

INGREDIENTS

Spray olive oil

4 (Four ounce) of rib eye steaks (trim small)

1/4 teaspoon offresh ground black pepper

1/2 teaspoon ofsalt

3 tablespoons of maple syrup

3 tablespoons of rosemary

3 tablespoons of fresh tarragon

3 tablespoons of chives or Mint or Rosemary or thyme or Sage Herbs (Any one that won't cause a trigger)

3 tablespoons of oregano (minced)

4 tablespoons of curly parsley

INSTRUCTIONS

1. Heat up your oven to 450 Degrees F and arrange a 12 inch non-stick pan into the oven.

2. Mix together the minced herbs and transfer to a plate. In another place, pour the maple syrup.

3. Sprinkle the steaks with salt and pepper, then coat the steak on both sides thoroughly in the maple syrup.

4. Rub coated steak in the minced herbs, turning gently until completely coated. Pat herbs in place, then repeat with each steak. Recoat steak if you have any leftover herbs or maple syrup.

5. Withdraw the skillet from oven and lightly spritz with oil, then add the steaks immediately to the hot skillet in other to sear well.

6. Place pan back into the oven and cook on the first side for about 4 minutes. Flip steak and cook for 6 minutes on the other side for rare.

Nutrition information per servings:
Calories: 241 kcal
Carbohydrates: 12g
Fat: 16g
Protein: 24g
Sodium 367mg

Pork Tenderloin

Prep time: 10 minutes
Cook time: 60 minutes
Servings: 6

INGREDIENTS

Spray olive oil
3/4 pounds of pork tenderloin (trimmed any excess fat)
1/2 cup of 2% milk
1/4 cup of low-fat sour cream
1 1/2 cups of low sodium chicken or vegetable broth
1/2 teaspoon ofsalt
1/4 cup of balsamic vinegar
1/2 cup of port
1/4 cup of dried cherries
1 minced clove garlic
1/4 cup of diced yellow onion
1 teaspoon of olive oil

INSTRUCTIONS

1. Heat olive oil over medium-high heat in sauce pan. Add in the onion with the garlic and cook without burning the garlic until tender.
2. Add the port, dried cherries, chicken stock and balsamic vinegar. Lower to medium heat and cook until sauce is reduced to about 1/2 cup and thick.
3. Transfer into your blender and process until you havea smooth mixture. Add milk and sour cream and blend again. Return back to the saucepan and heat through.
4. Heat up your oven to 425°F. Add the pork to a pan and transfer the pan into the hot oven then reduce heat to 375° Degrees.
5. Roast pork in the oven for 20 – 25 and checking until the internal temperature reaches 140°F – 145°F.
6. Remove roasted pork and allow to sit for about 5 minutes on the counter. Slice roasted pork into small medallions. Serve four oz. medallions with three tablespoons of the sauce.

Note: The sauce can also be made ahead and stored in the fridge. Add few tablespoons of water when reheating if the sauce is too thick. Onions may trigger GERD, but if they are cooked very well, they should be safe. You can decide to leave out or try green onions or shallots, they provide milder onion flavor, and you can try in small quantity.

Nutrition information per servings:
Calories: 208 kcal
Carbohydrates: 6g
Fat: 6g
Protein: 26g
Sodium 277mg

Roast Leg of Lamb

Prep time: 15 minutes

Cook time: 120 minutes

Servings: 8

INGREDIENTS

1 tablespoon of unsalted butter

1/2 cup of low sodium chicken broth

1 teaspoon of   olive oil

Fresh ground black pepper (to taste)

1/2 teaspoon ofsalt

3 tablespoons of fresh oregano

2 pounds of boneless leg of lamb (trim off excess fat and silver skin outside the leg)

INSTRUCTIONS

1. Heat up your oven to 325°F.

2. Sprinkle inner side of the lamb leg with pepper, oregano leaves and 1/4 teaspoon of the salt. Roll up the leg and truss with kitchen twine.

3. Add oil in a large pan over high-medium heat. Once it's hot, place the lamb and sear to brown on both sides.

4. Arrange the pan into the oven and roast the lamb about 45 minutes, turning at 15 minutes interval to brown both side. Check with a thermometer, it's done when it reads 145°F.

5. Remove from the oven and transfer onto a plate to rest.

6. Add the chicken broth in a skillet over medium-high heat. Pour the reserved salt and whisk until the sauce reduces by half. Add in butter and continue whisking until butter is melted. Slice lamb and serve with the sauce.

Nutrition information per servings:
Calories: 181 kcal
Carbohydrates: 0g
Fat: 9g
Protein: 23g
Sodium 222mg

Spaghetti and Meatballs

Prep time: 2 minutes

Cook time: 30 minutes

Servings: 2

INGREDIENTS

1 ounces of Parmigiano-Reggiano cheese (grated)

1 cups of tomato sauce (Some might be able to tolerate this without heartburn)

8 meatballs

8 ounces of spaghetti noodles

8 quarts of water

INSTRUCTIONS

1. Add water to large stockpot and boil over high heat. Once its boiling, add in the spaghetti noodles.

2. Meanwhile, add the meatballs with the tomato sauce in a large sauce pan and gently heat over medium heat. Once the sauce is heated through, reduce heat to low.

3. Once pasta is cooked, use tongs to remove the noodles and let them drain. Place the noodles in the sauce pan containing sauce and the meatballs and gently toss to combine. Serve immediately in bowl and top with the grated cheese.

Note:

The tomato sauce may contain GERD triggers and anyone with GERD may wish to avoid it.

Nutrition information per servings:

Calories: 464 kcal

Carbohydrates: 56g

Fat: 15g

Protein: 32g

Sodium 548mg

Pot Roast With vegetables

Prep time: 10 minutes

Cook time: 240 minutes

Servings: 6

INGREDIENTS

1 pounds of carrots (peeled and sliced thick)

2 pounds of small red potatoes (cut into large chunks)

2 medium onions (cut into wedges) (onions may trigger GERD, but if they are cooked very well, they should be safe. You can decide to leave out)

Fresh ground black pepper (to taste)

1 teaspoon of salt

1 tablespoon of dried sage

2 bay leaves

1 cup of water

2 pounds of bottom round (trimmed of excess fat)

2 teaspoons of olive oil

INSTRUCTIONS

1. Heat up your oven to 225°F.

2. Heat the olive oil over medium high heat in a medium stock pot or Dutch oven. Add in the bottom round.

3. Sear both sides of the meat, about 2 minutes on each side. Add a cup of water and withdraw from heat. Add the sage, bay leaves, onion, salt and pepper and stir.

4. Cover pot with a lid and transfer to the oven. Allow to roast for 3 hours.

5. Scoop out about half of the liquid and onions and add to a blender. Blend until smooth.

6. Add carrots and potatoes into the pot. Place pot back to the oven and cook for another 60 – 90 minutes.

7. Once time completes, remove roast and transfer onto a plate.

8. Pour the pureed liquid with onions into the pot and mix well to thicken. Serve topped with gravy.

Nutrition information per servings:
Calories: 381 kcal
Carbohydrates: 28g
Fat: 10g
Protein: 37g
Sodium 544mg

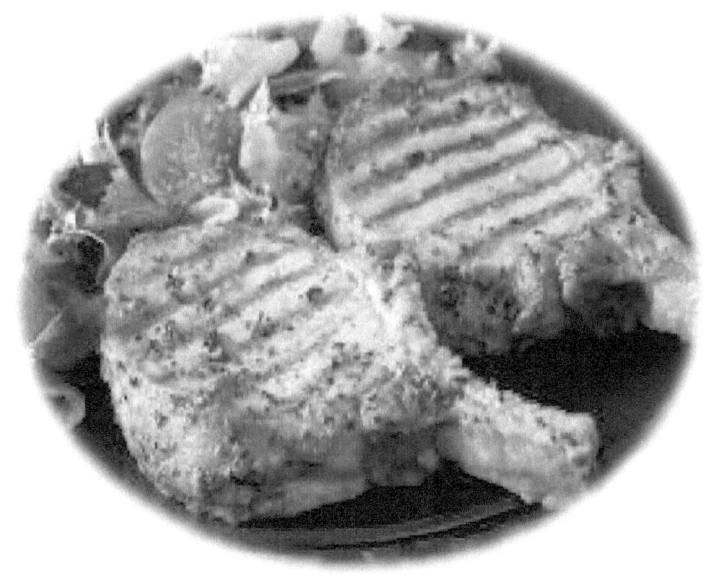

Mushrooms Pork Chops

Prep time: 8 minutes

Cook time: 30 minutes

Servings: 2

INGREDIENTS

8 oz of shiitake mushrooms (thinly sliced)

2 teaspoons of olive oil

2 (4 ounce) of pork chops

Fresh ground black pepper (to taste)

2 teaspoons of Chinese five spice powder

1 teaspoons of dark sesame oil

1 teaspoons of rice vinegar

1 teaspoons of honey

2 teaspoons of low sodium soy or gluten-free tamari sauce

1/3 cup water

INSTRUCTIONS

1. Mix the rice vinegar, honey, soy sauce, five spice powder, sesame oil and pepper together in a mixing bowl. Transfer to a ziplock bag.

2. Add the pork chops into the ziplock bag and leave to marinate overnight.

3. Once you are ready to cook, heat the olive oil over medium heat in a medium skillet. Add in the mushrooms and cook, stirring frequently for about 10 minutes until browned. Gather towards one side of the pan and place pork chops into the pan. Cover with the lid and cook for 10 minutes.

4. Flip pork chops, pour in water and continue cooking for more 5 minutes.

5. Transfer the pork onto a plate and let rest for about 2 minutes. Add 1 tablespoon of water at a timeif you notice the mushrooms are too dry. Serve the pork with mushrooms on top.

Nutrition information per servings:

Calories: 268 kcal

Carbohydrates: 12g

Fat: 11g

Protein: 27g

Sodium 244mg

Pork Chops Amana

Prep time: 10 minutes

Cook time: 30 minutes

Servings: 2

INGREDIENTS

2 (4 ounce) of center cut pork chops

1/4 cup of water

1/4 teaspoon of dried thyme leaves

1/4 cup of white wine (sweet like a Riesling)

1 tablespoon of balsamic vinegar

1 ounces of maple syrup

1/4 teaspoons of salt

2 teaspoons of sugar

2 medium granny smith apples, sliced (May trigger GERD for some people)

1 tablespoon of unsalted butter

INSTRUCTIONS

1. Heat the butter over medium-high heat in a medium sauté pan. Add the apples along with the sugar. Cook the apples about 20 - 25 minutes until apples are brown and caramelize but do not burn; stir periodically during the cooking period. Add the salt,

wine, balsamic vinegar, maple syrup with thyme leaves. Gently stir.

2. Heat up your oven to 400°F and arrange a medium skillet into the oven. Lower heat and let apples simmer on low heat for 10 minutes; stirring not too often. Add one tablespoon of water at a time if there is not enough liquid.

3. Once apples are cooked, lightly spritz the hot pan with oil and add in the pork chops. Transfer the skillet back into the oven and let cook for 8 to 10 minutes. Flip the pork chops and allow to cook for extra 8 to 10 minutes. Serve with mashed yams and top with caramelized apples.

Nutrition information per servings:
Calories: 345 kcal
Carbohydrates: 27g
Fat: 8g
Protein: 25g
Sodium 362mg

Pork Tenderloin with Mushrooms Barley

Prep time: 10 minutes

Cook time: 45-60 minutes

Servings: 4

INGREDIENTS

1/2 cup of water

2 cups of low sodium chicken or vegetable broth

1 pounds of pork tenderloin (cut into 1/2 inch cubes)

Fresh ground black pepper (to taste)

1 tablespoon of minced fresh sage

1/2 teaspoon ofsalt

1 cup of barley

1/2 large diced red bell pepper

1 pounds of sliced crimini mushrooms

1 large carrot (peeled and diced)

1 medium of diced onion

4 tablespoons of unsalted butter

INSTRUCTIONS

1. Heat up your oven to 325°F.

2. Heat the butter over medium heat in a medium Dutch oven or a large sauce pan. Add onion with the carrot. Cook, stirring frequently for about 5 minutes until the onion is tender.

3. Place mushrooms and cook, tossing constantly, until mushrooms are browned lightly.

4. Add the barley, red bell pepper,sage,pepper, pork and salt. Mix well and then add the water plus chicken stock. Stir.

5. Cover pot with the lid and transfer to the oven, checking every 14 minutes. If the liquid is not enough, add 1/4 cup water at a time as necessary until the barley is soft but not gummy for about 45 - 60 minutes.

Note: (Onions may trigger GERD, but if they are cooked very well, they should be safe. You can decide to leave out or try green **onions** or shallots, they provide milder **onion** flavor, and you can try in small quantity)

Nutrition information per servings:
Calories: 431 kcal
Carbohydrates: 42g
Fat: 9g
Protein: 35g
Sodium 494 mg

SOUP AND STEW RECIPES

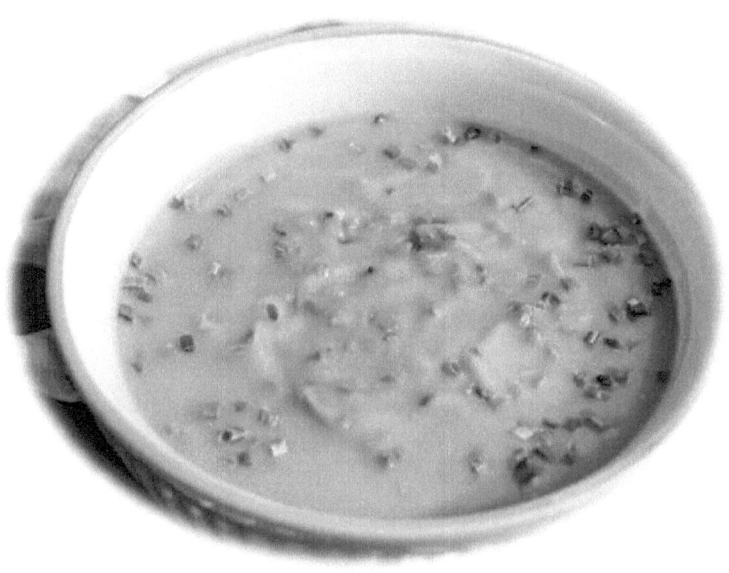

Scallions Carrots Miso Soup

Prep time: 15 minutes

Cook time: minutes

Servings: 4

INGREDIENTS

3 thinly sliced scallions

Pinch of wakame flakes

1/2 cup of extra firm tofu, cubed

1 cup of sliced carrots

Large handful of baby spinach

2 tbsp of miso paste (thinned out with a little water)

1 tbsp of toasted sesame seed oil

1 tbsp of Braggs amino acids or tamari

3 cups of water

3 cups of vegetable broth

2 cups of mushrooms, sliced

1/2 tsp of fresh ginger root, grated

1 tbsp of extra virgin olive oil

INSTRUCTIONS

1. Heat olive oil over medium-low heat in a large soup pot. Add fresh ginger and sauté until fragrant. Add in the mushrooms and cook until moisture is released.

2. Add in water plus broth and simmer for 30-45 minutes on low.

3. Turn heat off and withdraw the mushroom broth. Stir in toasted sesame seed oil and bragg's amino acids. Mix a little water with miso paste in a small bowl to thin it out then add to the soup.

3. Add carrots, spinach, wakame flakes and tofu into a bowl, and then pour steaming broth over the top. Garnish with sliced scallions and serve along with brown rice.

Nutrition information per servings:

Calories: 133 kcal

Carbohydrates: 9g

Fat: 9g

Protein: 5g

Sodium 327 mg

Vegan Fermented Vegetables

Prep time: minutes

Cook time: 15 minutes

Servings: 6-8

INGREDIENTS

A few sprigs fresh dill

2-3 tbsp of fine sea salt

1 quart of filtered water

6-8 organic pickling cucumbers cut to fit into jar

1 bag sliced organic radishes

1-2-lbs of organic carrots cut into sticks

INSTRUCTIONS

1. Prepare the brine by combining warm water with the salt and allow to cool.

2. Add enough fresh dill as needed.

3. Tightly add pickles, radishes and carrots into the jar, as many that can go in.

4. Once the brine is the cool pour into the jar, filling it to the top and making sure the vegetables are completely covered.

5. Lock the lid and allow to ferment for 7-14 days at room temperature for. Keep away from an area with high

temperature. Store leftover brine it in the refrigerator and used later.

Sweet Potato, Kale and Crumbled Tempeh Hash

Prep time: 10 minutes

Cook time: 30 minutes

Servings: 3

INGREDIENTS

2 tbsp of nutritional yeast

1/2 tsp of cayenne pepper

1/2 tsp of paprika

2 tbsp of apple cider vinegar

1/2 cup of crumbled organic tempeh

3 cups of chopped fresh kale

2 tbsp of extra-virgin olive oil, divided

1 medium unpeeled sweet potato, diced

1/4 tsp of black pepper

INSTRUCTIONS

1. Heat up your oven to 425°F.

2. Line aluminum foil over a 10-inch × 15-inch baking sheet.

3. In a small bowl, add the sliced potatoes plus one tbsp oil; toss to coat evenly.

4. Add the potatoes to the baking pan, spread and bake for about 20 minutes until potatoes are tender and outside crispy.

5. Heat the 1 tbsp of oil over medium-low heat in a large skillet. Add in the kale and sautéfor 2 minutes. Add in tempeh and cook for extra 1 more minute.

6. Pour the potatoes into pan, add cayenne pepper, vinegar, yeast and paprika. Cook, stirring constantly about 1–2 minutes, until incorporated. Add black pepper and serve warm.

Note: apple cedar of vinegar may be a trigger for some people, it's broadly accepted as safe to consume in a small measure.

Nutrition information per servings:
Calories: 180 kcal
Carbohydrates: 16g
Fat: 9g
Protein: 8g
Sodium 37 mg

Heartburn-Friendly Beef Stew

Prep time: 15 minutes

Cook time: 90 minutes

Servings: 6

INGREDIENTS

4 cups of water

1/8 teaspoon of ground allspice

1 1/2 pounds of red potatoes (peeled and 3/4 inch cubes)

2 bay leaves

1 pounds of carrots, sliced 1/4 inch thick)

1 tablespoon of Worcestershire sauce

1 tablespoon of fresh lemon juice

1 cup of white onion (sliced)

1/2 pounds of button mushrooms (quartered)

Cooking spray

1 1/2 pounds of flank steak (3/4 inch cubes)

1/4 teaspoon of fresh ground black pepper

1 teaspoon of salt

1/3 cup of all-purpose white flour

4 cups of water

INSTRUCTIONS

1. Pour water into a stock-pot and heat over high until it is at a shiver. Add onions and pearl and cook for 10 mins. Drain and transfer onions into a large stock pot.

2. Heat up your oven to 400°F. Mix the flour with pepper and salt inside a paper bag. Toss the flank steak cubes in the flour mixture until coated well.

3. Spritz a large cooking pan with cooking spray and place over high-medium heat. Add coated flank steak cubes (you can do in batches, make sure the pan is not over crowded) and cook,

stirring until brown on all sides. Once it's brown, transfer the meat into the stock pot.

4. Place the onions to pan and cook until onions are tender and brown; transfer to the stock pot.

5. Add the Worcestershire sauce with lemon juice to the pan, stirring constantly to deglaze the pan. Pour the liquid into the stock pot.

6. Add potatoes, carrots, allspice, bay leaves and water to the pot. Cover with the lid and place in the oven.

7. Allow to cook for an hour, gently stir each fifteen minutes interval.

Note:(Onions may trigger GERD, but if they are cooked very well, they should be safe. You can decide to leave out or try green onions or shallots, they provide milder onion flavor, and you can try in small quantity)

Nutrition information per servings:
Calories: 356 kcal
Carbohydrates: 37g
Fat: 8g
Protein: 30g
Sodium 544 mg

Mixed Butternut Squash Soup

Prep time: 5 minutes

Cook time: 60 minutes

Servings: 4

INGREDIENTS

1 cup of water

1/8 teaspoon of ground nutmeg

1/2 teaspoon ofdried thyme leaves

Fresh ground black pepper

1/2 teaspoon ofsalt

2 pounds of butternut squash

2 cups of water

INSTRUCTIONS

1. Set the steamer basket in a large sauce pan and heat 2 cups of water over high heat.

2. Arrange the squash cubes into the steamer basket; Steam about 20 - 30 minutes until soft. Allow to cool then place to the bottom of the saucepan with the remaining steaming water. Puree the squash and water using a stick blender or a blender until smooth.

3. Set the pan on the stove and heat on low, and add the thyme leaves, salt, ground nutmeg and pepper.

4. Gently reheat the soup. Add in water bit by bit until desired consistency is reached.

Nutrition information per servings:

Calories: 103 kcal

Carbohydrates: 27g

Fat: 0g

Protein: 2g

Sodium 300 mg

Chicken Celery and Black-Eyed Pea Soup

Prep time: 10 minutes

Cook time: 60 minutes

Servings: 4

INGREDIENTS

8 ounces of fresh spinach

2 15 ounce can of no salt added black eyed peas (drained)

2 cups of water

3 cups of low sodium chicken or vegetable broth

Fresh ground black pepper (to taste)

1/2 teaspoons of salt

1/2 teaspoons of dried thyme

2 teaspoons of dried sage

1 pounds of skinless boneless chicken thighs (cut into 1 inch cubes)

2 ribs celery (diced)

1 large diced red onion

1 teaspoon of olive oil

INSTRUCTIONS

1. Heat oil in a large skillet over medium heat. Add the celery and red onion and cook, stirring constantly until the onions is tender, about 5 – 7 minutes.

2. Add the chicken, thyme and sage and cook, stirring constantly about 5 – 7 minute until chicken is lightly browned.

3. Add in the black eyed peas, chicken stock, salt, pepper and water. Turn heat up and cook until soup starts to boil. Lower heat to medium-low and let soup simmers. Cook stirring not too often for about 40 minutes.

4. To serve, place 2 oz. of spinach in the bowl with 2 cups of soup.

Note: (Onions may trigger GERD, but if they are cooked very well, they should be safe. You can decide to leave out or try green onions or shallots, they provide milder onion flavor, and you can try in small quantity)

Nutrition information per servings:
Calories: 360 kcal
Carbohydrates: 3g
Fat: 8g
Protein: 38g
Sodium 509 mg

Lentil, carrots and Chickpea

Prep time: 10 minutes
Cook time: 75 minutes
Servings: 4
INGREDIENTS
Fresh ground black pepper to taste
3 bay leaves
1/4 teaspoon of salt
1 cup of water
3 cups of no salt added vegetable stock
4 oz. of peeled and diced carrots (about 2 medium carrots)
4 oz. of diced celery (about 3 stalks)
2 teaspoons of olive oil
4 oz. of dried chickpeas
4 oz. of dried lentils
2 quarts of water

INSTRUCTIONS

1. Place water in a large bowl, add chickpeas and lentils and allow to stand for up to an hours. Drain and rinse in water. Set aside.

2. Heat the oil in a large skillet over medium high heat. Add in the diced celery and cook, stirring frequently until slightly translucent. It should take about 4 minutes.

3. Add diced carrots and cook, stirring constantly for about 3 minutes.

4. Add the water, vegetable stock, lentils, chickpeas and bay leaves. Reduce to low medium heat and simmer for 45 minutes. Season with pepper and salt to taste and simmer for 15 more minutes. Serve.

Nutrition information per servings:
Calories: 202 kcal
Carbohydrates: 21g
Fat: 4g
Protein: 11g
Sodium 260mg

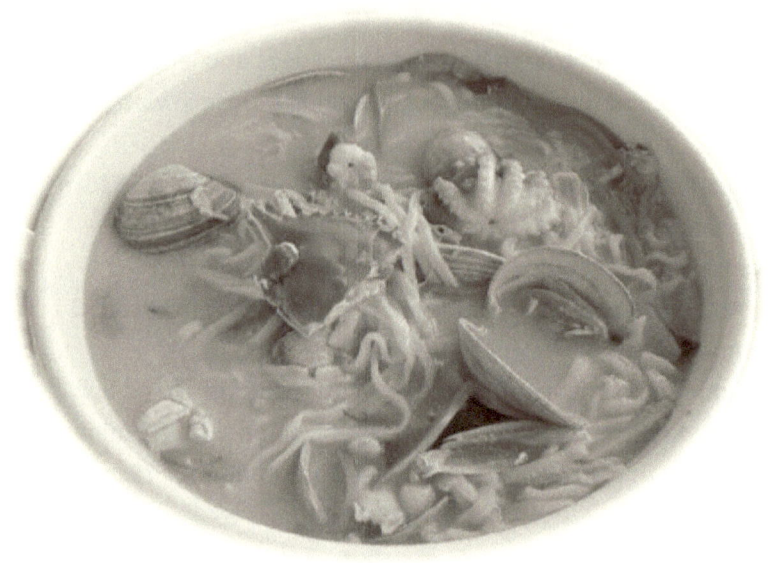

Speedy Potato Soup

Prep time: 10 minutes

Cook time: 30 minutes

Servings: 4

INGREDIENTS

1 green onion, sliced diagonally

4 oz. of reduced fat shredded)cheddar cheese

Fresh ground black pepper

1/4 teaspoon of salt

1/2 cup of 2% milk

5 cups of water

2 pounds of Idaho potatoes (cut into 1 inch cubes)

1 large diced white onion

1 teaspoon of olive or canola oil

INSTRUCTIONS

1. Heat olive oil in a large skillet over medium high heat. Add in the onion and cook, about 3 minutes, stirring frequently.
2. Stir in the potatoes plus five cups of water.
3. Turn heat up and cook until the water starts to boil and then lower heat to medium-low. Cook for 20 minutes until the potatoes are tender, stirring occasionally.
4. Remove from heat and allow the soup slightly cool. Let soup stand for 5 minutes, stir in the salt, pepper and milk.
5. Reheat the soup when ready to serve and garnish with one 1 ounce of cheddar cheese per serving

Note: (Onions may trigger GERD, but if they are cooked very well, they should be safe. You can decide to leave out or try green onions or shallots, they provide milder onion flavor, and you can try in small quantity)

Nutrition information per servings:
Calories: 268 kcal
Carbohydrates: 42g
Fat: 4g
Protein: 13g
Sodium 350mg

White Bean Turkey Soup

Prep time: 10 minutes

Cook time: 120 minutes

Servings: 8

INGREDIENTS

1 tablespoon of dried sage

Fresh ground black pepper (to taste)

3/4 teaspoon ofsalt

3 large peeled carrots (cut into large chunks)

3 large ribs celery (sliced thickly)

3 15 oz. can of no salt added white beans (drained and rinsed)

2 pounds of leftover turkey meat

Leftover turkey bones

2 quarts of water

INSTRUCTIONS

1. Heat water over high heat in a large stock pot and place the turkey bones, once the water starts to boil, reduce heat and allow to simmer for 30 minutes.

2. Strain the liquid and remove the bones. Add the broth, celery, carrots, turkey meat, whitebeans, pepper, sage and salt to the stock pot. Simmer for about 90 minutes over medium heat. Serve.

Nutrition information per servings:

Calories: 338 kcal

Carbohydrates: 17g

Fat: 5g

Protein: 42g

Sodium 311mg

Chicken Peas Egg Noodle Soup

Prep time: 10 minutes

Cook time: 25 minutes

Servings: 8

INGREDIENTS

4 cups of frozen peas

4 cups of diced, cooked skinless boneless chicken breasts

6 oz.(4 cups) uncooked egg noodles

1 tsp of salt

1 tsp of thyme

8 low-sodium chicken bouillon cubes

4 cups of carrots, peeled and chopped

4 quarts of water

4 cup of celery, trimmed and chopped

1 tbsp of olive oil

INSTRUCTIONS

1. Heat olive oil in a large pot over a medium-high heat. Add in the chopped celery and sauté for few minutes until translucent.

2. Add chicken bouillon cubes, water, chopped carrots, thyme, and salt. Cook until heated through.

3. Add the egg noodles to the pot. Stir together and bring to a boil. Turn heat down and cook until noodles are done, about 8 minutes.

4. Add the peas and cooked chicken breast. Return to a boil, lower heat to medium-low, cover and simmer for 5 to 10 minutes.

Nutrition information per servings:

Calories: 315 kcal

Carbohydrates: 33g

Fat: 7g

Protein: 29g

Sodium 737mg

Chicken Vegetable Cumin-Spiced Soup

Prep time: 10 minutes

Cook time: 60 minutes

Servings: 5

INGREDIENTS

1 cup of chopped kale

1 medium zucchini, spiralized

1 14-ounce can of white beans, rinsed

2 medium carrots, chopped

1/2 cup of barley

1/2 tsp of salt

8 cups of water

1 teaspoon dried oregano

1 tbsp of cumin

2 medium skinless, boneless chicken breast

INSTRUCTIONS

1. Heat water in a stock pot until its boiling, add in the chicken breast, oregano, cumin and 1/2 tsp of salt. Cook, covered about 15 minutes or until cooked through.

2. Remove chicken from pot and strain the liquid, reserving the liquid from cooking to use as base for soup.

3. Pour barley into the liquid and then bring to a boil. Cook with the lid on for about 20 minutes.

4. Meanwhile, shred the chicken with two forks. Set aside.

5. Add the white beans and carrots and cook for additional 10 to 15 minutes or until the carrots are a bit soft. Add in the shredded chicken, kale and zucchini. Simmer for additional 5 minutes and serve.

Nutrition information per servings:
Calories: 279 kcal
Carbohydrates: 33g
Fat: 2g
Protein: 22g
Sodium 436mg

Barley Beef Soup

Prep Time: 15 minutes
Cook Time: 1 hour 43 minutes
Servings: 10

INGREDIENTS

2 potatoes, soaked and diced
1 (16 ounces) package of vegetables, frozen
3 cups of water
1/4 cup of vegetable oil, divided
1/2 cup of barley
2 diced carrots
1 (14.5 ounces) can of chicken broth, low sodium
1/4 tsp of dried thyme
1/2 cup of sliced mushrooms
2 pounds of beef stew meat, diced into 1 inch cubes
1/2 tsp of black pepper

INSTRUCTIONS

1. Season the beef stew meat with black pepper.
2. Arrange the season beef into the pot, add 2 tbsp of oil to stew pot. Sauté for 5 minutes, add two extra tbsp of oil, add mushrooms and carrots.
3. Sauté for 5 more minutes, stirring frequently. Add thyme and sauté for three minutes.

4. Add water and broth into the pot, then add barley, potatoes and mixed vegetables. Stir and cook until heated through. Cover and simmer on low heat for1 to 1 1/2 hours

Nutrition information per servings:
Calories: 270 kcal
Carbohydrates: 22g
Fat: 2g
Protein: 23g
Sodium 105mg

Divine Potato Soup

Prep Time: 10 minutes
Cook Time: 40 minutes
Servings: 6 (1 1/2 cup each)
INGREDIENTS
1/2 cup of sour cream, fat free
4 oz of shredded Monterey jack cheese, reduce fat
1/2 tsp of pepper
4 cups of skim milk
1/3 cup of flour
2 large potatoes
INSTRUCTIONS
1. Place potatoes in the oven and bake at 400 degrees until tender.
2. When it's cool enough to handle, cut in half lengthwise and scoop the pulp out.
3. In a large sauce pan, add flour and slowly stir in milk, until well blended.

4. Add pepper and the scooped out potato pulp.

5. Cook, stirring frequently over medium heat until bubbly and thick.

6. Stir in the cheese until it's melted. Turn heat off and stir in sour cream.

Note:

Those that are lactose intolerant may avoid this recipe.

Nutrition information per servings:

Calories: 216 kcal

Carbohydrates: 29g

Fat: 1g

Protein: 15g

Sodium 272mg

FISH AND SEAFOOD RECIPES

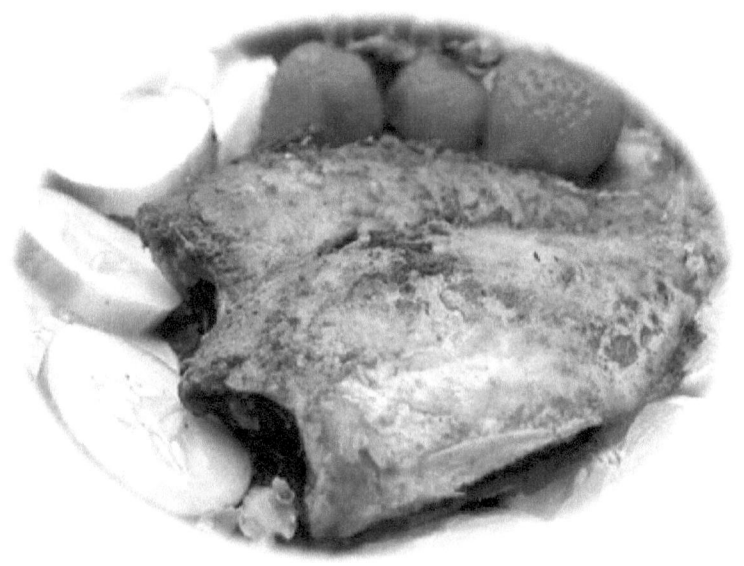

White fish Papaya

Prep time: 7 minutes

Cook time: 30 minutes

Servings: 2

INGREDIENTS

2 tablespoons of fresh cilantro leaves

4 tablespoons of water

1 teaspoon of corn starch

2 (6 ounce) of whitefish filets (tilapia,cod, orange roughly)

Fresh ground black pepper (to taste)

Spray olive oil

1/4 teaspoon of salt

1/4 cup of papaya juice

1 teaspoon of sesame oil

INSTRUCTIONS

1. In a small mixing bowl, whisk together the sesame oil, papaya juice, pepper and salt until well combined.

2. Heat a large non-stick frying pan over medium-high heat. Once pan is hot, lightly spray pan with olive oil. Place the fish filets and cook for 4 minutes, flip and cook the other side for another 4 minutes.

3. When it's one minute to the final cooking time, mix 4 tablespoons of water with the cornstarch in a small bowl until well mixed. Whisk the mixture into papaya sauce.

4. Pour papaya sauce into the frying pan containing the fish then flip once. Transfer the fish onto serving plates. Mix the sauce and spread on the fish. Top with a sprinkle of cilantro leaves. Serve and enjoy!

Nutrition information per servings:

Calories: 182 kcal

Carbohydrates: 6g
Fat: 3g
Protein: 30g
Sodium 384mg

Shrimp on Avocado Toast

Prep time: 5 minutes
Cook time: 5 minutes
Servings: 2

INGREDIENTS

1/4 mango, thinly sliced
Pinch of salt
1/2 medium avocado, mashed
2 slices of whole wheat bread
(Optional) 1 tsp of cilantro, finely chopped
1/8 tsp of cumin
1/2 tsp of lemon zest
1/2 tsp of olive oil
10 small shrimp or 8 medium shrimp, peeled and deveined

INSTRUCTIONS

1. Combine together the olive oil with shrimp, cumin, lemon zest and cilantro (optional) in a small bowl.

2. Place a small skillet on your stove and heat over medium. Add the seasoned shrimp and cook for 4 to 5 minutes, flipping midway.

3. Meanwhile, mash together the avocado with the salt and toast the bread slices.

Spread mashed avocado on top the toasted bread add mango slices to the top plus shrimp.

Note:
 Avocados may trigger heartburn but this recipe is a good stand-in for spreads. The secret is portion control.

Nutrition information per servings:
Calories: 177 kcal
Carbohydrates: 16g
Fat: 9g
Protein: 8g
Sodium 265mg

Cod With Potato Packets

Prep time: 5 minutes
Cook time: 5 minutes
Servings: 4
INGREDIENTS
8 slices of fresh lemon
1 or more teaspoon kosher salt
4 tsp of olive oil
2 tsp of dried thyme leaves
2 lbs of cod, divided into 8 pieces (Remove all skin from fish)
4 cups of sweet potato, julienned
INSTRUCTIONS
Heat up your oven to 400F.
1. Arrange 8 sheets of parchment paper and fold in half.
2. Gather 1/8 of sweet potatoes towards a side on the parchment and place a piece of cod on top.
3. Sprinkle each fish pieces with 1/8 tsp of thyme, 1 tsp olive oil, 1/8 tsp of salt and lastly top with a slice of lemon.

4. Fold the other half of the parchment paper over the fish, then fold and crease the edges of the pepper to form a closed and crescent shaped packet.

5. Place the packets onto the baking sheet and bake for about 20 minutes.

Withdraw from the oven and let cool for 5 minutes before removing the parchment paper. Serve

Nutrition information per servings:

Calories: 165 kcal;

Carbohydrates: 10g;

Fat: 5g;

Protein: 17g:

Sodium 934mg

Hearty Shrimp With Pasta

Prep time: 15 minutes

Cook time: 10 minutes

Servings: 4

INGREDIENTS

1/2 cup of grated Parmesan cheese

8 oz. of uncooked angel hair pasta

1 lbs of medium shrimp, peeled and deveined

1 tsp of dried oregano

1/2 tsp of salt

2 tsp of dried basil

1 tbsp of olive oil

Nonstick vegetable cooking spray

INSTRUCTIONS

1. Lightly spritz cooking spray over a large skillet. Heat olive oil in the skillet over medium-high heat for 1 to 2 minutes.

2. Add dried oregano, dried basil, shrimp and salt. Gently toss together to coat shrimp with ingredients.

3. Cook shrimps, turning once until its turning pink are cooked, about 6 to 8 minutes.

4. While the shrimps are cooking, cook the pasta the way instructed in the package directions. Drain.

5. Toss hot pasta with shrimp mixture and Sprinkle cheese on top and serve.

Nutrition information per servings:

Calories: 399 kcal

Carbohydrates: 49g

Fat: 9g

Protein: 28g

Sodium 1080 mg

Halibut Fillets with Cilantro

Prep time: 10 minutes
Cook time: 30 minutes
Servings: 2

INGREDIENTS

Fresh ground black pepper
2 (4 ounce) of halibut filets
1 tablespoons of low-sodium soy sauce
1/4 teaspoons of rice vinegar
2 tablespoons of fresh cilantro
1 tablespoons of peanut butter
3 tablespoons of unsalted butter

INSTRUCTIONS

1. Mix peanut butter with the butter, soy sauce, cilantro and vinegar; refrigerate. This can be prepared 12-24 hours ahead.
2. Heat up the oven to 425°F. Arrange a large pan in the oven.
3. Once the oven is hot, spray the pan lightly with oil. Sprinkle pepper on the halibut and transfer the filets into pan. Cook fillet in the oven about 5 minutes, flip and Cook for additional 7 to 10 minutes. To serve, top each fillet with half cilantro butter.

Note: Rice vinegar can be tolerated by most people and may not cause any trigger
Those that are lactose intolerant you make avoid this recipe.

Nutrition information per servings:
Calories: 246 kcal
Carbohydrates: 2g
Fat: 14g
Protein: 26g
Sodium 497 mg

Salmon LentilsWith Maple Marjoram Sauce

Prep time: 15 minutes

Cook time: 30 minutes

Servings: 2

INGREDIENTS

2 tablespoons of maple syrup

2 (4 ounce) of salmon filets

1 tablespoon of extra virgin olive oil

Fresh ground black pepper (to taste)

1 teaspoon of dried marjoram

1/4 teaspoon ofsalt

1/2 cup of low sodium chicken or vegetable broth

1 cup of water

1/2 cup of red lentils

2 medium peeled and diced carrots

1 large diced rib celery

Spray olive oil

INSTRUCTIONS

1. Lightly spray a medium skillet with olive oil. Place skillet over medium heat. Add the diced celery and diced carrots and cook for about 5 minutes, stirring constantly.

2. Stir in red lentils. Add the chicken stock, water, marjoram and salt; reduce heat to low simmer liquid. Cook, Stir occasionally until the lentils are just tender for about 20 - 25 minutes.

3. Once you are halfway into the cooking time, preheat your oven to 375°F. Set a skillet into the oven.

4. Once the lentils are cooked, add 1 tablespoon of olive oil, stir together and turn heat down.

5. Lightly spray the hot skillet with olive oil spray and place your salmon filets. Add 1 tbsp maple syrup and cook for about 4 minutes.

6. Flip salmon over and top with the remaining tbsp maple syrup. Cook for additional 4 - 6 minutes.

7. Top cooked salmon with cooked lentils and the sauce remaining at the bottom of the skillet on top the salmon.

Nutrition information per servings:

Calories: 512 kcal

Carbohydrates: 33g

Fat: 18g

Protein: 38g

Sodium 434 mg

Tuna Rotini Pasta Mushroom Soup Casserole

Prep time: 7 minutes

Cook time: 30 minutes

Servings: 6

INGREDIENTS

Spray cooking oil

2 ounces of Parmigiano-Reggiano (grated)

1/8 teaspoon ofground nutmeg

Fresh ground black pepper (to taste)

1 (16 ounce) bag of frozen peas

2 (6 ounce) cans of light tuna packed in water, Drain (no salt added)

1/4 cup of 2% milk

2 cans of Cream of Mushroom Soup (Campbell's Healthy Request)

16 ounces of whole wheat or gluten-free rotini pasta

3 quarts of water

INSTRUCTIONS

1. Heat up the oven to 375°F.
2. Boil water over high heat in a medium stock pot add cook pasta for 10 minutes in the boiling water. Drain.
3. Meanwhile, place the milk, mushroom soup, drained tuna, nutmeg, pepper and peas in a large bowl. Gently mix together.
4. Add hot pasta in the mushroom/tuna mixture and gently stir.
5. Lightly spritz an oblong pan (12 inch) with oil. Place the pasta/tuna mixture in the pan and carefully press down using a rubber spatula. Sprinkle top with cheese and transfer the pan to the oven. Bake in the oven for 20 minutes.
Note:
Those that are lactose intolerant you make avoid this recipe.

Nutrition information per servings:
Calories: 512
Carbohydrates: 65g
Fat: 7g
Protein: 33g
Sodium 665 mg

Oven Seared Halibut Fillets

Prep time: 5 minutes
Cook time: 30 minutes
Servings: 2

INGREDIENTS

Spray olive oil
1/4 cup of extra virgin olive oil
1/2 cup of fresh basil leaves
2 4 ounce of halibut filets (rinse in cold water, pat dry)
1/4 teaspoon of salt
Fresh ground black pepper

INSTRUCTIONS

1. Process the basil with olive oil in a blender and blend until mixture is smooth.
2. Heat up your oven to 425°F and arrange a medium skillet in the oven.
3. Meanwhile, place the skin side of halibut filets up on a cutting board; cut a slight slits in the skin about quarter inch apart. Sprinkle side facing up with pepper and salt.
4. Spray the hot skillet lightly with oil. Transfer halibut filets in the skillet with skin side down.
5. Place skillet in the oven and cook for 10 - 13 minutes. To serve, place fish skin side up and spread 1 1/2 tsp of basil oil on top.

Nutrition information per servings:
Calories: 183 kcal
Carbohydrates: 0g
Fat: 9g
Protein: 23g
Sodium 351 mg

Trout With Pecans

Prep time: 15 minutes

Cook time: 30 minutes

Servings: 2

INGREDIENTS

1 teaspoon of unsalted butter

1/4 cup of white wine

1 tablespoon of olive oil

2 4 ounce of boneless trout filets (skin on)

1 tablespoon of maple syrup

1/4 teaspoon of smoked paprika

Fresh ground black pepper to taste

1/8 teaspoon of salt

1 1/2 teaspoon of fresh rosemary

1 tablespoon of fresh sage

1 1/2 ounces of raw pecans

INSTRUCTIONS

1. Pulse the 6 to 11 ingredients in a blender or mini-chopper until the consistency resemble that of coarse sand. (The pecans size should be smaller than dried lentils.)

2. In a small bowl, place the mixture and add in maple syrup. Gently mix until well blended.

3. Preheat the oven to 375F and place a large skillet. Place the trout fillet on a cutting board or plate with skin side down. Rub the flesh side of the trout evenly with pecan mixture.

4. Once the pan is hot, remove pan and add olive oil then place back to the oven to heat oil for a minute. Remove and arrange the trout skin side down in the skillet, place back in the oven to cook for 5 minutes.

5. Set the broil function on the oven. Broil fish until the crust is a bit browned, about 3-5 minutes.

6. Withdraw from the oven and transfer the trout to a plate.

7. Place the skillet over medium-high heat on the stove. Add white wine to the skillet, swirling for 35-45 seconds, and then place the butter. Stir well until butter is melted. Spread the sauce over the trout filets to serve.

Nutrition information per servings:

Calories: 445 kcal

Carbohydrates: 9g

Fat: 31g

Protein: 26g

Sodium 206 mg

Salmon PeasMac and Cheese

Prep time: 10 minutes
Cook time: 60 minutes
Servings: 4

INGREDIENTS

Fresh ground black pepper (to taste)
1/4 teaspoon ofsalt
1 cup of frozen peas
8 ounces of skinless salmon (sliced into thin strips)
4 ounces of grated Monterey Jack cheese (reduced-fat)
1/4 teaspoon of dried tarragon
1/2 cup of 2% milk
2 large eggs
8 ounces of whole wheat or penne pasta or shells (gluten free)
4 quarts of water

INSTRUCTIONS

1. Heat up your oven to 325°F.
2. Bring water to boil over high heat in a medium stock-pot. Add pasta and cook for few minutes until the pasta is slightly cooked, chewy but not tough.
3. Meanwhile, in a medium mixing bowl, combine the milk with eggs and whisk until well blended.
4. Add the salmon, tarragon, peas, cheese, pepper and salt to the bowl and gently mix.
5. Once pasta is done, drain and stir into the salmon/cheese bowl until well blended.
6. Transfer pasta mixture to a 9 inch Pyrex dish and bake in the preheated oven for 30 minutes. Allow to slightly cool before serving.

Nutrition information per servings:
Calories: 463 kcal
Carbohydrates: 42g
Fat: 15g
Protein: 35g
Sodium 421 mg

CHICKEN AND POULTRY RECIPES

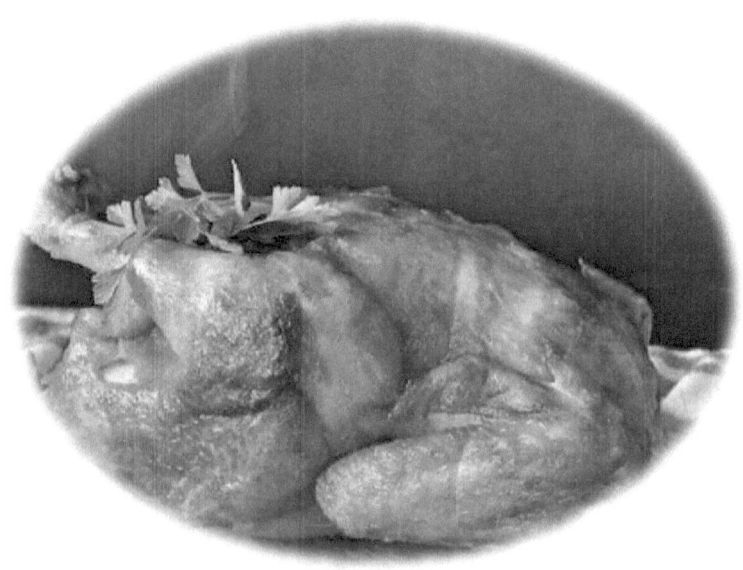

Breaded Chicken Nuggets

Prep time: 20 minutes
Cook time: 20 minutes
Servings: 4

INGREDIENTS

1 1/4 cups of riced cauliflower (buy pre-riced or make your own)
1/2 cup of plain breadcrumbs
1/2 tsp of kosher salt
1/2 tsp of garlic powder
1 large egg
1 lbs of skinless, boneless chicken breast, cut into 1 by 2 inch rectangles

INSTRUCTIONS

1. Heat the oven to 350F.
2. Line a large baking sheet with parchment paper, set aside.
3. Combine together the egg, salt and garlic powder in a small shallow plate, whisk until well combined.
4. Combine the cauliflower and breadcrumbs in a separate plate.
5. Dredge chicken pieces in the first bowl containing the egg mixture. Allow any excess to drip off. Then coat the chicken in the cauliflower and breadcrumbs mixture (pat to make it adhere).
6. Transfer the coated chicken pieces to the lined baking sheet and bake for 20 minutes, flip once halfway through cooking.

Nutrition information per servings:
Calories: 331 kcal
Carbohydrates: 10g
Fat: 5g
Protein: 30g
Sodium 483 mg

30-Minute Chicken With Fennel And Turmeric

Prep time: 5 minutes

Cook time: 25 minutes

Servings: 4

INGREDIENTS

4 medium skinless, boneless chicken breasts

¼ tsp of kosher salt

½ tsp of ground fennel seed

1 tsp of ground turmeric

2 tsp of olive oil

INSTRUCTIONS

1. Heat the oven to 375F.

2. Line a large baking tray with parchment paper.

3. Mix fennel, turmeric, oil and salt in a small bowl. Place the chicken and let it marinate for at least one hour or overnight. (If you have time to do so)

4. Alternatively, place the chicken in the prepared baking tray and spray with oil mixture.

5. Place in the oven and bake until the internal temperature reaches 160F, about 20 to 25 minutes. Let it slightly cool before slicing and serving.

Nutrition information per servings:

Calories: 158 kcal

Carbohydrates: 0g

Fat: 5g

Protein: 26g

Sodium 207 mg

Chicken Livers With Tuscan Risotto

Prep time: 15 minutes

Cook time: 30 minutes

Servings: 2

INGREDIENTS

1/2 ounce of grated Parmigiano-Reggiano

8 ounces of chicken livers

Fresh ground black pepper (to taste)

1/4 teaspoon ofsalt

1 teaspoon of dried sage (crush with the fennel)

3 cardamom seeds (shell removed and crushed with the fennel)

1 teaspoon of fennel seed (crushed into powder)

4 cups of water

1 large shallot, chopped

1/2 cup of arborio rice

2 teaspoons of olive oil

INSTRUCTIONS

1. Heat the oil in a sauce pan over medium high heat.

2. Add shallot and cook, stirring regularly until the shallot is slightly tender.

3. Add the risotto; cook, stirring frequently for about 1 minute.

4. Add the cardamom, water, sage, fennel and salt. Stir and simmer on low heat. Cook stirring periodically until tender and almost done but not mushy.

5. Add the chicken livers and pepper. Add extra water if needed, a bit at a time. Cook Stirring occasionally for 8 to 10 minutes or until the chicken liver is slightly browned. Top with the parmesan and serve.

Nutrition information per servings:

Calories: 404 kcal
Carbohydrates: 48g
Fat: 9g
Protein: 27g
Sodium 493 mg

Chicken Shallot with Cranberry Sauce

Prep time: 5 minutes
Cook time: 30 minutes
Servings: 2

INGREDIENTS

1 4 ounce of skinless, boneless chicken breast (per serving)
2 teaspoon of unsalted butter
Fresh ground black pepper (to taste)
1/4 teaspoon of salt
1 cup of water
1/4 cup of white wine
1 cup of dried sweetened cranberries
1 large minced shallot
Spray olive

INSTRUCTIONS

1. Grease a medium frying pan with oil spray over medium heat. Add the minced shallot and cook stirring constantly until shallot is soft.
2. Divide the dried cranberries into 4, reserve a portion and stir in the remaining three. Cook for 5 minutes. Add the water with wine. Stir and simmer on low heat. Add the salt and pepper to the simmering sauce and cook for about 15 minutes until slightly soft.

3. Puree sauce in a mini-chopper or blender and strain through a fine mesh sieve.

4. Transfer back to the pan and add the reserve cranberries. Cook about 15 minutes on low heat and add butter, swirl until melted. If the sauce is too thick add more water.

5. Preheat to 375° and Place a large pan. Once the pan is hot, lightly spray the pan with oil. Add the chicken breasts. Place back to the oven and cook for 5-6 minutes.

6. Remove pan from the oven, turn chicken breasts over to sear the other side.

Cook for 15 minutes, turn the chicken just once. Top with sauce to serve.

Nutrition information per servings:

Calories: 258 kcal

Carbohydrates: 27g

Fat: 4g

Protein: 27g

Sodium 223 mg

Turkey Skewers

Prep time: 10 minutes

Cook time: 30 minutes

Servings: 4

INGREDIENTS

Spray olive oil

Fresh ground black pepper (to taste)

1/2 teaspoon of salt

2 tablespoons of fresh rosemary

2 tablespoons of extra virgin olive oil

16 ounces of skinless, boneless turkey breast (slice into 16 strips)

INSTRUCTIONS

1. Pierce 2 turkey breast strips with wooden skewers.

2. Mix together the rosemary, olive oil, salt and pepper. Pour mixture in a zip lock bag and add the turkey skewers, close and place the ziplock bag in the refrigerator overnight.

3. Heat a lightly greased skillet over medium-high heat and place the skewers.

Cook for 15 – 20 minutes 5 turning occasionally.

Nutrition information per servings:

Calories: 184 kcal

Carbohydrates: 0g

Fat: 7g

Protein: 28g

Sodium 346 mg

Chicken Quinoa Stuffed Veggie Roll-Ups

Prep time: 15 minutes

Cook time: 40 minutes

Servings: 4

INGREDIENTS

Zest from 1/2 lemon

2 tbsp of feta cheese, crumbled

1/2 cup of chopped spinach

1/4 tsp of oregano, dry

1/4 tsp of salt

2 medium skinless, boneless chicken breasts, pound to 1/4 inch thickness

1/4 cup of broccoli stalks, julienned

1/2 medium carrot, julienned

2 tbsp of dry quinoa

INSTRUCTIONS

1. Cook quinoa the way instructed in the package directions.

2. Steam the broccoli stalks and carrots until slightly soft.

3. Heat up the oven to 350F and place the chicken on a parchment paper lined baking sheet and spray lightly with olive oil; rub on both sides with salt.

4. Fill the middle of the chicken breasts with vegetables, quinoa, oregano, lemon zest, spinach and cheese. Keep the filling from reaching the edges.

5. Roll the stuffed chicken breast from one to the other. Insert toothpicks on either end or tie with twine to keep secure.

6. Heat a small pan over medium heat and place the stuff chicken rolls, heat for about 5 minutes until golden brown on all sides.

7. Place the rolls into the baking tray, place in the oven and cook about 15 minutes or until cooked through. Allow to cool for 5 minutes before slicing.

Nutrition information per servings:

Calories: 112 kcal

Carbohydrates: 5g

Fat: 3g

Protein: 15g

Sodium 413 mg

Breaded Chicken Parmesan

Prep time: 15 minutes

Cook time: 45 minutes

Servings: 4

INGREDIENTS

4 chicken breasts, boneless, skinless, pat dry

1/2 cup of seasoned bread crumbs

3 tbsp of grated good-quality Parmesan cheese

Dash of Italian seasoning

Dash of salt

4 tsp of olive oil

INSTRUCTIONS

1. Preheat the oven to 375 F.

2. Spray a baking dish lightly with cooking spray.

3. Combine together the bread crumbs, Parmesan cheese, Italian seasoning, and salt in a small bowl. Mix to combine.

4. Place the chicken breasts on a plate and coat with olive oil.

5. Dip chicken in the bread-crumb mixture; make sure both sides are coated. Place in the baking dish and sprinkle the chicken with any remaining breadcrumb mixture.

6. Place in the oven and bake for 35 to 45 minutes (uncovered) or until it's done.

Nutrition information per servings:
Calories: 331 kcal
Carbohydrates: 9g
Fat: 19g
Protein: 29g
Sodium 721 mg

Chicken Veggies Pie

Prep time: 15 minutes
Cook time: 40 minutes
Servings: 4
INGREDIENTS
1 cup of biscuit mix
3/4 cup of skim milk, divided into 1/2 cup and 1/4 cup
1 (14.75-oz.) can of cream-style corn
1 cup of frozen peas, thawed
1 cup of frozen carrots, thawed
1 tbsp of olive oil
1/2 tsp of salt
1 lbs of skinless, boneless chicken breasts (cut into 1-inch cubes)
INSTRUCTIONS
1. Preheat your oven to 400 F.
2. Season the chicken breasts cubes with 1/2 teaspoon salt.
3. Heat the oil in a sauce pan over medium-high heat. Add the chicken cubes and cook stirring occasionally for 8 minutes or

until browned. Add 1/4 cup skim milk and cream style corn.
Cook, stirring until bubbly and thickened.

4. In a 3-quart baking dish, place the chicken and add carrots and peas.
Cover and bake for about 25 minutes.

5. Meanwhile, combine together the biscuit mix and reserved skim milk. Stirring until it forms a soft dough. Take the baking dish out of the oven and uncover.

6. Spoon the biscuit/milk mixture over the baked chicken mixture and spread to cover.

7. Bake in the oven uncovered until golden brown for about 10 minutes.

Nutrition information per servings:
Calories: 430 kcal
Carbohydrates: 43g
Fat: 12g
Protein: 34g
Sodium 1077 mg

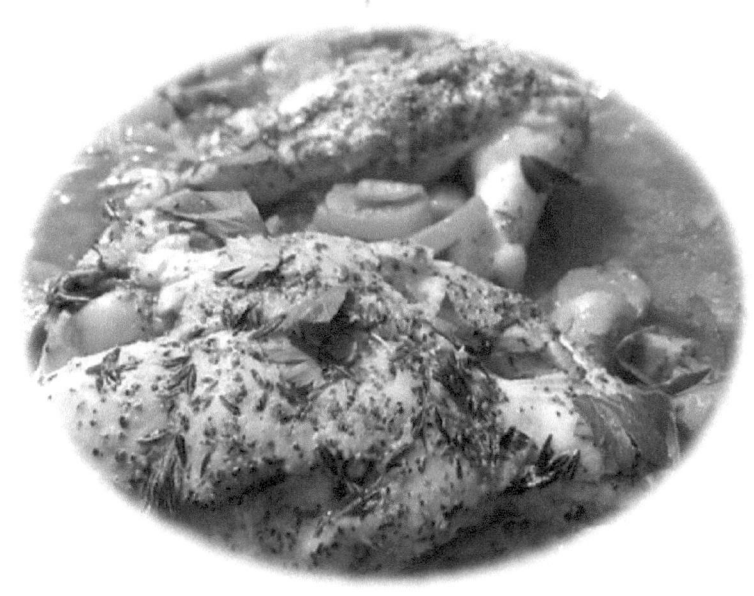

Chicken Edamame With Noodles

Prep time: 10 minutes

Cook time: 30 minutes

Servings: 2

INGREDIENTS

2 tablespoons of dry roasted unsalted peanuts

Slivered red onion to taste

1 small shredded carrot

4 ounces of whole wheat or gluten-free spaghetti

1/2 cup of frozen edamame (soybeans)

6 ounces of skinless, boneless chicken breast, cut in strips)

1/8 teaspoon ofred pepper flakes

2 tablespoons of low sodium chicken or vegetable broth

2 teaspoons of low-sodium soy sauce

1/2 of lime juice
1/4 cup of fresh cilantro leaves
3 tablespoons of smooth peanut butter
3 quarts of water

INSTRUCTIONS

1. Place chicken stock, soy sauce, lime juice, cilantro, red pepper flakes and peanut butter in a blender and blend until smooth. Set aside.

2. In large saucepan, add 3 quarts water over high heat. Once the water starts boiling, reduce to medium heat until water starts to simmer. Place the chicken strips and cook for about 5 minutes.

3. Remove chicken from the pan and increase the heat until water returns to a boil. Add spaghetti. Cook until almost al dente, about 8-10 minutes. Add soybeans and cook for extra 1 minute.

4. Drain the edamame and pasta but reserve 1/2 cup of the liquid. Return edamame and Pasta to sauce pan. Reduce to medium heat and add chicken, peanut sauce, onions and shredded carrots, toss to combine well. (Leave out the onions if it is a GERD trigger for you).

5. The sauce may be too thick for you, add reserved liquid from pasta to thin the sauce, 1 tbsp at a time. Top serve top with peanuts.

Note:

Those that are sensitive to gluten may wish to avoid this recipe

Nutrition information per servings:
Calories: 581 kcal
Carbohydrates: 49g
Fat: 23g

Protein: 44g

Sodium 257 mg

Chicken Skewer with Peanut Sauce

Prep time: 10 minutes

Cook time: 30 minutes

Servings: 6

INGREDIENTS

Spray olive oil

1/4 cup of cilantro leaves

1/8 teaspoons of salt

1/2 teaspoons of low sodium soy or gluten-free tamari sauce

6 tablespoons of low sodium chicken broth

1/4 cup of smooth peanut butter

12 wooden skewers of toothpicks

1 1/2 pounds of skinless, boneless chicken breast (cut into 2 ounce strips)

3 teaspoons of sesame oil

3 tablespoons of fresh minced ginger

INSTRUCTIONS

1. Pierce skewers through the chicken strips.

2. Combine together the sesame oil with minced ginger in a large zipper bag and place the chicken skewers. Allow to marinate for up to 4 hours or overnight.

3. Place the chicken stock, peanut butter, cilantro, soy or gluten-free tamari sauce and salt in a blender. Process until smooth, then store in the refrigerator to chill.

4. One you have finished marinating, heat a large skillet over high heat, once hot, reduce to medium high heat and spritz with olive oil.

5. Remove the chicken from the marinade and place on the skillet. Cook for 5 minutes. Turn-over and cook for 8 to 12 minutes more. Top with the peanut sauce.

Nutrition information per servings:

Calories: 138 kcal

Carbohydrates: 0g

Fat: 3g

Protein: 26g

Sodium 84 mg

Heartburn Friendly Fried Chicken

Prep time: 10 minutes

Cook time: 30 minutes

Servings: 6

INGREDIENTS

4 (4 ounce) skinless boneless chicken breasts

1/4 teaspoon of cayenne pepper

1/4 teaspoon of garlic powder

1 tablespoon of Dijon mustard

1/2 teaspoon of ground black pepper

1 teaspoon of dried thyme

1/2 teaspoon of dried oregano

1 teaspoon of dried rosemary

1 (5 ounces) box of plain melba toast

1 large egg white

Spray oil

1 large egg

1/4 teaspoon of salt

INSTRUCTIONS

1. In a small mixing bowl, place the Dijon mustard, egg, with the egg white. Whisk until mixture is smooth.

2. Place the oregano, rosemary, thyme, melba toast, garlic powder, cayenne pepper black pepper and salt in a food processor and process into small breadcrumbs. Some of the pieces should be about the size of currants.

3. Heat up the oven to 400°F. Dip each chicken breast in the mustard/egg mixture. Allow any excess to drip. Coat in the breadcrumbs mixture, turn and pat until well coated.

4. Transfer the coated chicken onto a baking rack or cookie sheet and bake in oven for 3 minutes. Then lightly spray chicken on top

with the oil. Bake for 5 more minutes and then flip. Lightly spray again with the oil, bake for more 6 minutes.

Note:

Those that are sensitive to gluten may avoid this recipe

Nutrition information per servings:
Calories: 293 kcal
Carbohydrates: 8g
Fat: 4g
Protein: 33g
Sodium 588 mg

SALADS AND VEGETARIAN RECIPES

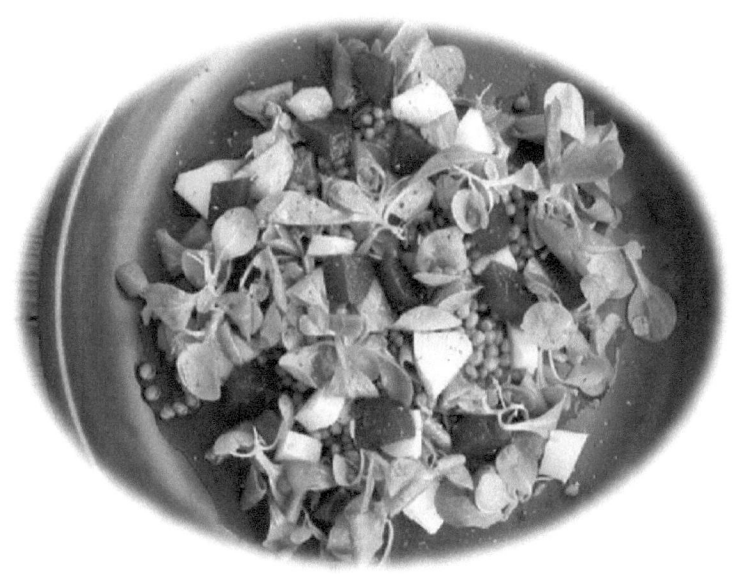

Pan Grilled Vegetables

Prep time: 10 minutes

Cook time: 10 minutes

Servings: 6

INGREDIENTS

1 large zucchini, sliced lengthwise

1 bunch asparagus, trim ends

1 bell pepper, remove ribs and seeds, the cut into large pieces

1 medium peeled eggplant, slice lengthwise

2 tbsp of chopped fresh oregano

1 tbsp of rice vinegar

½ tsp of kosher salt

1 tbsp of olive oil

INSTRUCTIONS

1. Whisk together the chopped oregano, vinegar, olive oil and salt in a large bowl.

2. Place zucchini, bell pepper and eggplant into bowl and toss with marinade until well coated.

3. Heat a grill pan to medium-high or outdoor grill. Place the vegetables over grill. Cook for about 4 minutes per side. Gently toss asparagus on grill and cook for 3 to 4 minutes until tender. Serve cooked vegetables warn on a large platter.

Nutrition information per servings:

Calories: 74 kcal

Carbohydrates: 6g

Fat: 3g

Protein: 3g

Sodium 9 mg

Lighter Avocado Chicken Salad

Prep time: 10 minutes

Cook time: 30 minutes

Servings: 4

INGREDIENTS

1/2 cup of diced celery (about 1 rib)

Freshly cracked pepper

1/4 tsp of garlic powder

2 tbsp of plain nonfat Greek yogurt

1 small avocado, mashed

Freshly cracked black pepper

Garlic powder, to taste

1 large chicken breast shredded to about 2 cups

INSTRUCTIONS

1. Heat up your oven to 350F. Season the chicken thoroughly with pepper and garlic powder.

2. Arrange seasoned chicken breast into a baking dish and cover with foil.

3. Place in the oven and bake for 25 to 35 minutes. It's done when you insert a thermometer in the center and it reads 165F. Remove chicken from the baking dish, allow cooling before you shred.

4. Smash the avocado in a large bowl. Stir in yogurt, garlic powder with the pepper. Add the shredded chicken and celery. Place in an airtight container and refrigerate.

Note:

Avocados may trigger heartburn though, but the secret is portion control.

Nutrition information per servings:

Calories: 174 kcal;

Carbohydrates: 6g

Fat: 7g

Protein: 23g

Sodium 362mg

Noodles Salad

Prep time: 10 minutes

Cook time: 10 minutes

Servings: 8

INGREDIENTS

1/3 cup of nonfat plain Greek yogurt or fat free sour cream

3 tbsp of real or light mayonnaise

Freshly ground pepper to taste and as tolerated

1/4 tsp of salt

2 tsp of parsley flakes (or 2 tbsp of fresh parsley, finely chopped

2 cups of dry whole wheat macaroni noodles

3 hard-boiled eggs

Optional Additions: (if tolerated):

1/4 cup finely chopped celery

1/4 cup finely chopped sweet or dill pickles

INSTRUCTIONS

1. Boil your eggs if you haven't done this already. Cook the macaroni noodles as instructed in the package directions, about 8 minutes. Drain well then rinse in cold water. Allow to cool.

2. In serving bowl, place the noodles, parsley, pepper and salt to taste, with any other additional ingredients as tolerated.

3. Blend together the Greek yogurt with mayonnaise in small bowl, then mix into in bowl containing the noodles.

4. Peel the eggs and scoop out half of the yolks then Chop the rest and mix with the macaroni mixture.

5. Place in an airtight container and refrigerate overnight for few hours or overnight.

Nutrition information per servings:
Calories: 129 kcal
Carbohydrates: 22g
Fat: 2.4g
Protein: 6g
Sodium 142 mg

Broccoli and Blue Cheese Salad

Prep time: 10 minutes
Cook time: 30 minutes
Servings: 2
INGREDIENTS
1 ounces of blue crumbled cheese (This is gluten free)
1 tablespoon of pine nuts
1 large bunch broccoli stalk (cut flowerets from stalks)
1 quart of water
INSTRUCTIONS
1. Fit a steamer basket onto a medium saucepan, pour in water and heat over high, bring to a boil.
2. Place the broccoli and steam for about 8 minutes.
3. Meanwhile, toast the pine nuts over medium-high heat in a small skillet, shaking constantly for about 5 minutes.
4. Once broccoli has finished steaming, shake broccoli to remove water and add to large bowl.
5. Add the pine nuts and blue cheese immediately and gently mix together until blue cheese is melted. Chill in the refrigerator before serving.

Note:
Those that are lactose intolerant may wish to avoid this recipe.

Nutrition information per servings:
Calories: 130 kcal
Carbohydrates: 8g
Fat: 7g
Protein: 8g
Sodium 250 mg

Heartburn Friendly Mango Coleslaw

Prep time: 20 minutes
Cook time: minutes
Servings: 2

INGREDIENTS

1 cup of diced fresh mango
1 cup of grated carrots
4 cups of shredded green cabbage
½ tsp of kosher salt
½ tsp of celery seed
2 tsp of sugar
1 tbsp of canola or avocado oil
¼ cup of rice vinegar

INSTRUCTIONS

1. Whisk together the canola or avocado oil, vinegar, celery seed, sugar and salt in a large bowl.
2. Add carrots, cabbage, and mango. Toss together to coat well with the dressing.

3. Let rest for 10 minutes at room temperature before serving or cover and chill in the refrigerator about 12 hours before serving.

Nutrition information per servings:
Calories: 64 kcal
Carbohydrates: 8g
Fat: 3g
Protein: 1g
Sodium 216 mg

Mushroom Salad

Prep time: 30 minutes
Servings: 2
INGREDIENTS
2 leaves Romaine lettuce
8 ounces of white mushrooms slice very thin
1/2 teaspoon of fresh orange zest
Fresh ground black pepper (to taste)
1/8 teaspoon of salt
2 tablespoon of 2% milk
2 tablespoon of reduced fat sour cream
2 teaspoons of apple cider vinegar
2 teaspoons of coarse ground mustard
1 tablespoon of olive oil
INSTRUCTIONS
1. Whisk together the mustard, sour cream, olive oil, milk, vinegar, pepper and salt. Add fresh orange zest. Chill in the refrigerator.

2. Toss the thinly sliced mushrooms together with the dressing and serve over romaine leaf.

Nutrition information per servings:
Calories: 122 kcal
Carbohydrates: 6g
Fat: 10g
Protein: 5g
Sodium 227 mg

Chilled Vegetable Quinoa Salad

Prep time: 10 minutes
Cook time: 5 minutes
Servings: 2

INGREDIENTS

1 cup of asparagus spears, cut into 3-inch pieces
1/2 cup of fresh or frozen peas
1 cup of cooked quinoa
2 cups of arugula
1/2 cup of radishes, sliced thinly
1/4 cup of fresh roughly chopped basil leaves
1 tbsp of olive oil
1/2 tsp of freshly cracked black pepper

INSTRUCTIONS

1. Place the peas and asparagus in a small saucepan. Add water and bring to a gentle boil. Cook about 1 minute until asparagus are bright green. Remove from heat without delay. Place peas and asparagus in an ice water bath so it will stop cooking. Drain.

2. Toss the peas and asparagus, radishes, arugula, basil and quinoa in a large bowl.

Whisk the olive oil, and pepper together in a small bowl. Pour dressing on top of the salad and toss to finely coat. Chill in the refrigerator until ready to serve.

Nutrition information per servings:
Calories: 265 kcal
Carbohydrates: 28g
Fat: 10g
Protein: 5g
Sodium 46 mg

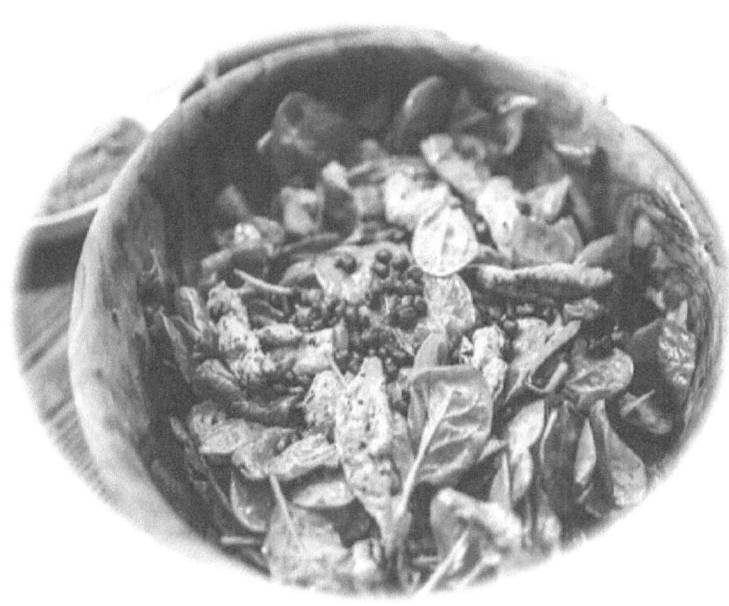

Special Waldorf Salad

Prep time: 10 minutes

Cook time: 30 minutes

Servings: 8

INGREDIENTS

1 1/2 teaspoon of honey

1/4 cup of low-fat sour cream

1/4 cup of low-fat mayonnaise

1/4 cup of raisins

1/4 cup of coarsely chopped walnuts

1 cup of celery (dice large)

1 tablespoon of fresh lemon juice

1 medium red delicious apple cored

2 medium granny smith apples, cored

INSTRUCTIONS

1. Cut the apples into 1/4 inch cubes with the fresh lemon juice.

2. Add raisins, celery and walnuts .Toss to coat.

3. Add sour cream, mayonnaise and honey. Carefully mix until finely blended.

4. Place in the refrigerator to chill for up to 2 hours before serving.

Note:

Those that are lactose intolerant may wish to avoid this recipe.

Nutrition information per servings:

Calories: 123 kcal

Carbohydrates: 16g

Fat: 6g

Protein: 1g

Sodium 75 mg

Basil Farro/Quinoa Salad

Prep time: 10 minutes

Cook time: 30 minutes

Servings: 8

INGREDIENTS

Pinch freshly cracked black pepper

1 minced clove garlic

1 tbsp of balsamic vinegar

1 tbsp of olive oil

1/3 cup of fresh mozzarella (in small balls, halved, cubed)

1/2 cup of fresh basil leaves, thinlysliced

1 cup of cherry tomatoes, halved (Might be a trigger for some)

3 cups of farro or quinoa

INSTRUCTIONS

1. Cook the farro or quinoa according to package instructions.

2. Combine together the farro or quinoa, basil, tomatoes, and mozzarella in a large bowl.

3. Whisk the remaining ingredients together in a small bowl. Pour dressing over faro or quinoa and toss to coat. Serve right away or cover and chill in the refrigerator up to 2 days.

Nutrition information per servings:

Calories: 406 kcal

Carbohydrates: 57g

Fat: 10g

Protein: 17g

Sodium 148 mg

Black beans Zucchini Salad

Prep time: 5 minutes

Servings: 4

INGREDIENTS

1/2 tsp of salt

1/2 lemon zest

2 tbsp of dill, chopped

1 cup of black beans

1 cup of green peas

2 medium zucchini

INSTRUCTIONS

1. Cut the zucchini into ribbons using a vegetable peeler

2. In a small bowl, combine together all of the ingredients. Chill in the refrigerator before serving.

Nutrition information per servings:

Calories: 95 kcal

Carbohydrates: 18g

Fat: 1g

Protein: 6g

Sodium 387 mg

Potato ` Salad

Prep time: 10 minutes

Cook time:60 minutes

Servings: 6

INGREDIENTS

2 teaspoons of paprika

Fresh ground black pepper to taste

1/4 teaspoons of salt

4 tablespoons of reduced-fat mayonnaise

1 – 5 ounceof no salt added canned tuna in water, drain

1 cup of frozen peas (thawed)

2 large hard boiled eggs (cut into small dice)

8 oz. carrots (peeled and dice into 1/4 inch)

1 lbs of Yukon Gold

3 quarts of water

INSTRUCTIONS

1. Bring water to a boil in a large skillet over high heat.

2. Place the diced carrots and cook until carrots are tender, about 15 minutes. Remove and set aside.

3. Add Yukon Gold potatoes into the hot water and let it simmer for 30 minutes. Remove the potatoes and set aside to cool on the counter for 10 minutes, then chill in the refrigerator.

4. Peel off the skin from the potatoes. Cut the potatoes into 1/2 inch cubes.

5. In a mixing bowl, place cube potatoes, carrots, tuna, peas, eggs, mayonnaise, paprika, salt and pepper. Gently fold together and chill in the refrigerator before serving.

Nutrition information per servings:

Calories: 153 kcal

Carbohydrates: 17g

Fat: 3g
Protein: 11g
Sodium 336mg

Cheesy Mac and Cheese

Prep time: 5 minutes

Cook time:45 minutes

Servings: 4

INGREDIENTS

Fresh ground black pepper

1/8 teaspoon of salt

5 ounces of grated cheddar cheese (reduced-fat)

1/2 cup of 2% milk (1 % milk will work)

2 large eggs

8 ounces of penne pasta (whole wheat or gluten-free)

4 quarts of water

INSTRUCTIONS

1. Bring water to a boil in a medium stock-pot over high heat. Add in the pasta and cook until al dente. Drain once it's done.

2. Meanwhile, combine together the milk with eggs, add to a medium sauce pan and whisk until smooth. Add the grated cheese and salt.

3. Add drained pasta to the pot and cook over medium heat. Stir constantly until cheese is melted. Make sure the mixture does no boil. Once the sauce is thick enough remove from the heat. Stir in the black pepper to taste and serve immediately.

Nutrition information per servings:

Calories: 306 kcal

Carbohydrates: 45g

Fat: 6g
Protein: 21g
Sodium 344mg

Fettuccine Alfredo

Prep time: 10 minutes
Cook time: 30 minutes
Servings: 2
INGREDIENTS
1 tablespoon of minced parsley
4 ounces of fettuccine (whole wheat or gluten-free)
4 quarts of water
1 ounceof grated Parmigiano-Reggiano
1 ounceof semi-soft goat cheese
3/4 cup of 2% milk (chilled)
2 teaspoon of all-purpose white flour
2 roasted cloves garlic (minced)
1 teaspoon of extra virgin olive oil
INSTRUCTIONS
1. In a medium non-stick skillet, heat the olive oil over medium heat and cook roasted garlic slowly, stirring constantly without browning the garlic. If the garlic is brown, it will be bitter.
2. Slowly add in the flour and cook, Stir frequently for about 1 minute until well blended and the mixture resemble coarse corn meal. Do not allow the mixture to brown.
3. Slowly whisk in the cold milk making sure no clumps forms until sauce starts to thicken and its smooth.
4. Add the goat cheese with a whisk until melted and smooth. Add the Parmigiano-Reggiano and whisk until melted and the sauce becomes creamy. Turn heat down to the lowest.

5. Add water in a large pot and bring to a boil. Add the whole wheat or gluten-free fettuccine and cook about 12 – 15 minutes until just tender. Drain.

6. Add the pasta to the sauce, toss well to coat. Sprinkle top with the parsley and serve.

Nutrition information per servings:

Calories: 389 kcal

Carbohydrates: 47g

Fat: 12g

Protein: 20g

Sodium 377mg

Chickpea Lentil Soup

Prep time: 10 minutes

Cook time: 75 minutes

Servings: 4

INGREDIENTS

3 bay leaves

1 cup of water

3 cups of no salt added vegetable stock

2 medium carrots (4 oz) of carrots (peeled and diced)

3 (4 oz) of diced celery stalks

2 teaspoons of olive oil

4 oz of dried chickpeas

4 oz of dried lentils

2 quarts of water

Fresh ground black pepper to taste

1/4 teaspoon ofsalt

INSTRUCTIONS

1. Add 2 quarts of water in a large bowl, add the chickpeas and lentils. Let stand for up to 10 hours. Drain chickpeas and lentils, rinse and set aside.
2. In a large sauce pan, place the olive oil over medium high heat. Add diced celery, cook stirring constantly for 4 minutes until slightly soft and translucent.
3. Add diced carrots, cook and Stir frequently for about 3 minutes.
4. Add 1 cup of water, vegetable stock, chickpeas with lentils and bay leaves. Turn heat down to medium low and simmer for about 45 minutes. Season with pepper and salt and simmer for extra 15 minutes. Serve.

Nutrition information per servings:
Calories: 202 kcal
Carbohydrates: 21g
Fat: 4g
Protein: 11 g
Sodium 206 mg

Roasted SquashWith lettuce Zucchini Tacos

Prep time: 10 minutes

Cook time: 45 minutes

Servings: 4

INGREDIENTS

2 cups of shredded lettuce

4 oz of reduced-fat shredded Monterey Jack cheese

2 tablespoon of pumpkin seeds (pepitas)

1 tablespoon of olive oil

Fresh ground black pepper (to taste)

1/8 teaspoon of salt

1 teaspoon of molasses

2 teaspoon of cocoa powder

1 teaspoon of ground oregano

1 teaspoon of ground cumin

2 small zucchini

2 small yellow squash

INSTRUCTIONS

1. Slice the zucchini and squash lengthwise into 4 and cut each lengths in half. (It should give you about 3-4 inches length).

2. Place a large skillet in the oven and heat to 325°F.

3. In a bowl, place the molasses, oregano, cumin, cocoa powder, salt and pepper. Blend with a rubber spatula until incorporated. Place squash slices and toss together well to coat.

4. Pour olive oil into the hot skillet, add pumpkin seeds, zucchini and squash.

5. Roast for about 15 minutes. Tossing constantly.

6. Place the cooked squash mix in the taco shells and add lettuce and shredded cheese on top.

Nutrition information per servings:

Calories: 441 kcal

Carbohydrates: 11g

Fat: 31g

Protein: 27 g

Sodium 486 mg

Vegetables AndCheese Frittata

Prep time: 10 minutes

Cook time: 30 minutes

Servings: 6

INGREDIENTS

1/4 cup of crumbled goat cheese

1/8 tsp of turmeric

4 large eggs

1 tbsp of olive oil

1/4 tsp of salt

1 tsp of oregano

1/2 tsp of thyme

1 tsp of basil

1/2 cup of sliced baby bella mushrooms

1/2 small diced sweet potato

1 medium diced carrot

1/2 cup of small broccoli florets

1/2 medium diced zucchini

INSTRUCTIONS

1. Heat up the oven to 350F.

2. Greased a 9-inch cake pan. Add the mushrooms, sweet potato, carrots, broccoli florets and zucchini to the pan and toss with

olive oil, oregano, basil, thyme and salt. Roast until the carrots and sweet potato are softened, it takes about 15 to 20 minutes.

3. While the vegetables are cooking, whisk together crumbled goat cheese, eggs and turmeric in a small bowl.

4. Open the oven and remove the vegetables. Evenly spread the vegetables throughout the pan.

5. Spread the egg/cheese mixture on top the vegetables and cook until the eggs are set, it takes about 5 to 10 minutes. Withdraw from oven and allow cooling before Slicing.

Nutrition information per servings:
Calories: 110 kcal
Carbohydrates: 4g
Fat: 7g
Protein: 7 g
Sodium 190 mg

SIDE DISH

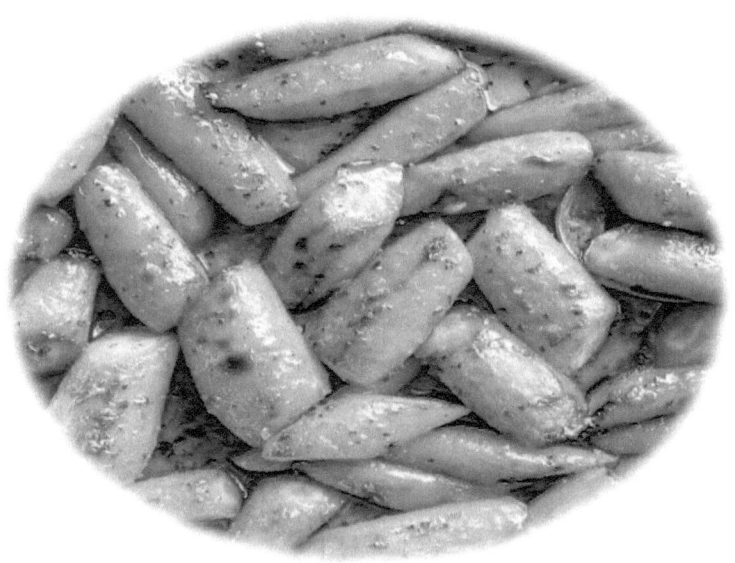

Spotty Carrots

Prep time: 5 minutes

Cook time: 30 minutes

Servings: 2

INGREDIENTS

1/4 teaspoon ofsalt

1 tablespoon of maple syrup

1 teaspoon of unsalted butter

8 oz of carrots

2 cups of water

INSTRUCTIONS

1. Arrange a steamer basket fitted in a pot, add the water and boil over high heat. Steam until the carrots are slightly soft, it should take about 10 -15 minutes.

2. Combine together the butter, cooked carrots, salt and maple syrup until well combines and serve.

Nutrition information per servings:

Calories: 89 kcal

Carbohydrates: 15g

Fat: 2g

Protein: 1 g

Sodium 224 mg

Creamy Peas

Prep time: 5 minutes

Cook time: 30 minutes

Servings: 2

INGREDIENTS

1 ounce of reduced fat cream cheese

1 teaspoon of coarse ground mustard

Fresh ground black pepper (to taste)

1/8 teaspoon of dried tarragon

A pinch of salt

2 tablespoons of water

1 1/3 cup of frozen peas

INSTRUCTIONS

1. Place water, peas, tarragon, salt and pepper in a small skillet over medium high heat.

2. Cook, stirring occasionally for about 5 minutes until most of the water is evaporated; lower heat to medium. Add the cream cheese and mustard and cook until the cheese is melted, about 3 minutes. Serve.

Nutrition information per servings:

Calories: 119 kcal

Carbohydrates: 17g

Fat: 2g

Protein: 7 g

Sodium 243 mg

Easy Pizza Dough

Prep time: 5 minutes

Cook time: 90 minutes

Servings: 4

INGREDIENTS

2 1/2 cups of all-purpose flour

1 teaspoon of sugar

1 teaspoon of dry active yeast

1/2 teaspoon of salt

1 cup of warm water

INSTRUCTIONS

1. Heat water to about 110°F to 115°F in the microwave. To get the accurate heat level, you can use a thermometer. It is very important the water is not too hot or it will kill the yeast, let it just be warm to touch

2. In a large mixing bowl, add sugar and yeast and then add the warm water into the mixture, stirring frequently until well mixed. Leave the mixture to stand for 5 - 7 minutes until it's foamy.

3. Combine together all-purpose flour and salt into the yeast mixture and mix with a fork to form coarse dough. Mix dough with your hand until well blended and a dough ball is formed.

4. Place the dough in a bowl, cover the bowl and place in a sink. Add hot water to the bottom, about 4 inches to the bottom. The heat coming from the hot water will help the dough rise.

5. Leave the dough to rise to double its original size, about 30 – 40 minutes. Punch the dough with your finger a couple of times and allow rise another 30 minutes.

6. When it's done rising, remove from the bowl and slice into 4 equal sizes. Preserve the dough that you are not using immediately by covering in plastic wrap and chill.

Note:

Those that are gluten sensitive may wish to avoid this recipe.

Nutrition information per servings:
Calories: 231 kcal
Carbohydrates: 59g
Fat: 1g
Protein: 8 g
Sodium 293 mg

Oven Toast Yam Fries
Prep time: 10 minutes
Cook time: 30 minutes
Servings: 4
INGREDIENTS
Spray olive oil
1/2 teaspoon of no salt added Cajun spice blend
Fresh ground black pepper (to taste)
1/8 teaspoon of salt
2 (5 ounces each) small yams
INSTRUCTIONS
1. Place a large pan in the oven and heat up to 325°F.
2. Wash the yams properly and slice into wedges.
3. When the oven is hot, spray the pan lightly with oil.
4. Place yam wedges in the hot pan and sprinkle top with cajun spice, salt and pepper. Spray top lightly with the olive oil.
5. Place pan back to the oven and cook, tossing frequently for about 25 minutes. Serve immediately.

Nutrition information per servings:
Calories: 199 kcal

Carbohydrates: 35g
Fat: 3g
Protein: 2 g
Sodium 194 mg

Creamy Cauliflower Lentils

Prep time: 5 minutes
Cook time: 45 minutes

Servings: 4
INGREDIENTS
Fresh ground black pepper (to taste)
1/2 teaspoon of salt
1/2 cup of light coconut milk
2 medium heads of cauliflower (cut into small florets)
2 cups of water
1 cup of black lentils
3 cups of water
INSTRUCTIONS
1. In a medium sauce pan, add 3 cups of water over high heat.
Bring to a boil and add in the black lentils, stir well and reduce to
low heat.
2. Cook on low heat about 20 to 25 minutes or until the water is
evaporated and lentils are soft. If water completely evaporates
before the lentils are soft, add a little more water.
3. Meanwhile, place a steamer basket in a medium stock pot,
add two cups of water over high heat. Add the cauliflower florets
and steam until soft, about 20 – 25 minutes.

4. Puree the cauliflower until smooth using a stick blender or a blender. Add coconut milk, pepper and salt, and puree.
5. Gently stir the lentils into the puree. Serve immediately.

Nutrition information per servings:
Calories: 256 kcal
Carbohydrates: 22g
Fat: 3g
Protein: 18 g
Sodium 381 mg

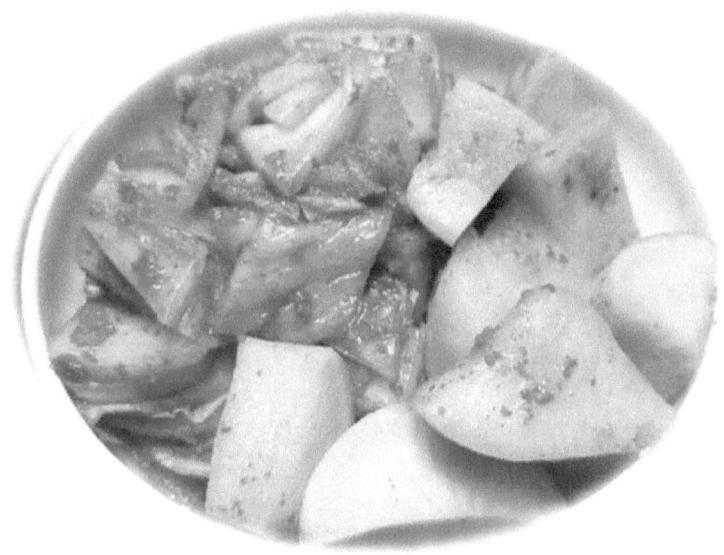

Oven Baked Crispy Fries

Prep time: 10 minutes

Cook time: 40 minutes

Servings: 4

INGREDIENTS

1/4 tsp of freshly ground black pepper

1/2 tsp of kosher salt

1 tbsp of olive oil

4 medium russet potatoes

INSTRUCTIONS

1. Heat the oven to 400F.

2. Wash the potatoes thoroughly to remove any dirt.

3. Slice lengthwise into evenly sized slices with the skins on.

4. Transfer into a parchment paper lined baking sheet.

5. Drizzle top with the olive oil and add salt and pepper.

6. Gently toss to evenly blend with the seasoning.

7. Place in the oven and bake for about 35-40 minutes, toss the French fries once or twice until golden and crisp. Remove and leave to slightly cool before serving.

Nutrition information per servings:

Calories: 194 kcal

Carbohydrates: 37g

Fat: 4g

Protein: 4 g

Sodium 449 mg

Buttermilk Mashed Potatoes

Prep time: 10 minutes

Cook time: 30 minutes

Servings: 4

INGREDIENTS

1 tablespoon of fresh ginger

1/4 teaspoon of salt

1/3 cup of 2% milk

1/3 cup of non-fat buttermilk

1 teaspoon of unsalted butter

1 pounds of Yukon Gold potatoes (Cut in quarter)

2 quarts of water

INSTRUCTIONS

1. Add the potatoes in a large stock pot filled with water over high-medium heat. The water should cover potatoes with about an inch. Once the water starts boiling, reduce heat until the water is simmering.

2. Cook the potatoes until the middle is slightly tender, about 15 – 20 minutes. Turn heat off and remove the pot. Drain.

3. Add in the milk, buttermilk, butter, grated ginger and salt. 4. Mash together until smooth and creamy. You can leave some chunks if you prefer. But do not mash too smooth so it won't turn pasty potatoes. To taste add ground black pepper.

Nutrition information per servings:

Calories: 107 kcal

Carbohydrates: 18g

Fat: 2g

Protein: 4 g

Sodium 186 mg

Log Shape Biscuits Rounds

Prep time: 10 minutes

Cook time: 40 minutes

Servings: 4

INGREDIENTS

2/3 cup of non-fat buttermilk

3 tablespoons of unsalted butter

1/4 teaspoon of salt

1 teaspoon of baking powder

1/2 teaspoon o f baking soda

1 cup of whole wheat flour

1 cup of all-purpose flour

INSTRUCTIONS

1. Heat up your oven to 325°F.

2. Place a medium sized mixing bowl under a sifter. Sift the flour and whole wheat, baking powder and baking soda into the bowl.

3. Add in butter and mix using a fork until well blended. Add the buttermilk and fold into the flour mixture with a rubber spatula until a fine dough forms. Work together using your hands until a dough ball forms.

4. Transfer dough ball onto a cutting board and roll into a large log shape. Cut dough log into eight biscuit rounds.

5. Transfer to a non-stick cookie sheet, place in the oven and bake for about 12 - 15 minutes.

Nutrition information per servings:

Calories: 135 kcal

Carbohydrates: 22g

Fat: 3g

Protein: 4 g

Sodium 358 mg

Porcini Cornmeal bread

Prep time: 10 minutes

Cook time: 4 minutes

Servings: 8

INGREDIENTS

1 tablespoon of porcini and truffle oil

1/4 teaspoons of baking soda

3 teaspoons of baking powder

1 tablespoon of Worcestershire sauce

3 tablespoon of honey

2 large eggs

1/2 cup of brown rice flour

1 1/2 cups of reduced-fat buttermilk

1 1/4 cup of coarse ground yellow cornmeal

1 ounceof dried porcini mushrooms

INSTRUCTIONS

1. Blend dried porcini mushrooms into a fine dust using a spice grinder or a blender.

2. Heat up the oven to 400°F.

3. Mix the cornmeal with the porcini dust in a mixing bowl and mix in the buttermilk until well mixed. Allow to stand for 20 minutes.

4. In a small bowl, place the Worcestershire sauce, eggs and honey and whisk until frothy.

5. In another small bowl, Place the baking powder, brown rice flour and baking soda, blend well using a fork.

6. In a 10-inch cast iron skillet, add the oil and transfer the pan into the oven.

7. Add the wet ingredients mixture and rice mixture into the cornmeal mixture, stirring until mixed well.

8. Take the skillet out of the oven and add the oil to the batter. Mix well until well blended.

9. Transfer the batter to the hot pan and transfer to the oven. Bake for about 25 minutes. Allow the pan to cool before slicing.

Nutrition information per servings:
Calories: 200 kcal
Carbohydrates: 36g
Fat: 4g
Protein: 7 g
Sodium 261 mg

Spinach With Artichoke Dip

Prep time: 15 minutes

Cook time: 30 minutes

Servings: 16

INGREDIENTS

1/8 teaspoon of ground nutmeg

1/4 teaspoon of salt

1 ounceof reduced-fat cream cheese

2 1/2 ounces of grated mozzarella cheese

1/2 cup of fat-free mayonnaise

2 (10-ounce) packages of frozen spinach, thawed

2 (15 ounce) can of artichoke hearts, packed in water

INSTRUCTIONS

1. Drain and press out all the liquid from the spinach into a bowl through a sieve. Reserve the liquid for later use.

2. Drain artichoke and place with the nutmeg, spinach, salt, cream cheese, mayonnaise and mozzarella in a food processor;

Process a few seconds until almost smooth. Pour in liquid from the spinach, one tbsp at a time until smooth.

3. When ready to serve, Transfer the dip in a heatproof bowl. Place bowl in the microwave in 30 second intervals, stirring thoroughly in between each interval. The heat should be able to melt the cheese and add make it creamy. It shouldn't be too hot so not to overcook the spinach. Serve and enjoy.

Nutrition information per servings:
Calories: 41 kcal
Carbohydrates: 3g
Fat: 2g
Protein: 3 g
Sodium 201 mg

DESSETS RECIPES

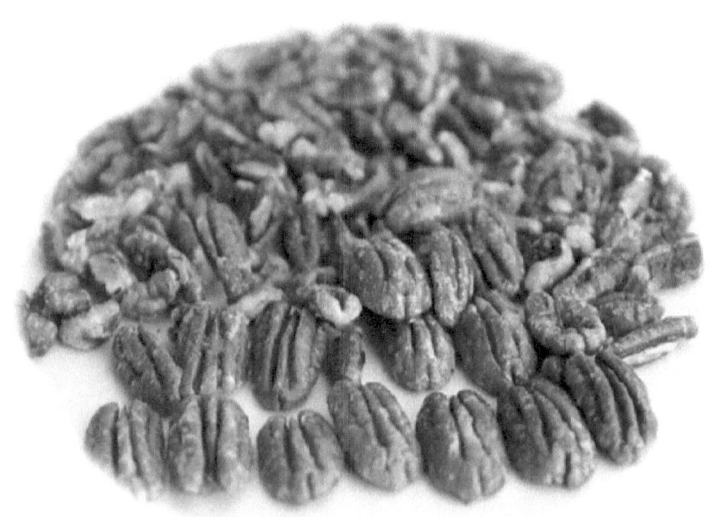

Milder Apple Crisp

Prep time: 25 minutes

Cook time: 30 minutes

Servings: 6

INGREDIENTS

6 tbsp of 100% apple juice

1/3 cup of slivered almonds or crunch with chopped pecans

1/2 tsp of kosher salt

2 tbsp of light brown sugar (packed)

1.2 cup of rolled oats

2 tbsp of all-purpose flour

3 tbsp of unsalted butter (cold, diced)

2 tbsp of sugar

1/4 tsp of lemon zest (freshly grated)

1/2 lemon, juiced

1 tsp of cinnamon

1 tsp of cornstarch

4 medium apples (peel and diced)

INSTRUCTIONS

1. Heat up the oven to 350F.

2. Line a baking sheet with parchment paper. Spritz 6 ramekins with nonstick cooking spray and place over the baking sheet.

3. Mix together the apples, cinnamon, cornstarch, lemon zest, lemon juice, and sugar in a medium bowl. Toss together and let it rest for 10 minutes.

4. In a another bowl, mix together the oats, flour, butter, brown sugar, almonds and salt; mix until well combined.

5. Evenly spread the apple mixture into the ramekins, sprinkle the top with the topping. Add a tbsp of apple juice on each.

6. Bake in the oven until golden and bubbly, about 30 minutes. Withdraw from the oven and let cool a bit before serving.

Nutrition information per servings:
Calories: 197 kcal
Carbohydrates: 24g
Fat: 10g
Protein: 2 g
Sodium 197

Easy Prep Strawberry Sorbet

Prep time: 5 minutes

Cook time: 60 minutes

Servings: 4

INGREDIENTS

1 pound of fresh strawberries (stemmed)

1/3 cup of sugar

1/2 cup of water

INSTRUCTIONS

1. In a small sauce pan, combine the sugar with water over medium high heat.

2. Once the water starts boiling, whisk until the sugar is dissolved. Cook for 1 minute more, whisking. Turn heat off.

3. Set aside and allow to cool for about 5 minutes.

4. Place the strawberries with the sugar solution in a blender and blend until mixture is smooth. Pulse in ten second bursts for a minute.

5. Transfer the mixture into an airtight container. Freeze and whisk the mixture Every 7 to 10 minutes vigorously. Once the mixture starts to thicken, change to rubber spatula to freeze completely. Serve.

Nutrition information per servings:
Calories: 100 kcal
Carbohydrates: 23g
Fat: 0g
Protein: 1 g
Sodium 1

Strawberries Almond Parfait

Prep time: 30 minutes
Servings: 4
INGREDIENTS
4 teaspoon of agave for serving
1/4 cup of toasted almonds (sliced)
2 cups of strawberries (sliced)
1/4 cup of chia seeds
1/8 teaspoon of kosher salt
1 teaspoon of vanilla
2 tablespoons of agave
1 cup of Greek yogurt (plain low fat)
1 cup of unsweetened vanilla almond milk
INSTRUCTIONS
1. Place the vanilla almond milk, vanilla, agave, Greek yogurt and salt in a medium bowl. Gently whisk until well blended.
2. Add in the chia seeds, blend and allow to sit for 25 minutes. Stir well, cover, and place in the refrigerator overnight.
3. When ready to serve, Combine the agave and the strawberries slices, toss to coat stir in the almonds.
4. In a sturdy glasses or glass parfait dishes, add the pudding and layer with the berry mixture.

Nutrition information per servings:

Calories: 199 kcal

Carbohydrates: g

Fat: 7g

Sodium 197

Rice With Coconut Pudding

Prep time: 5 minutes

Cook time: 10 minutes

Servings: 6

INGREDIENTS

1/2 teaspoon of ground ginger

1/4 cup of shredded coconut

2 cups of cooked rice

1 (1 ounces) package of instant sugar free, fat free vanilla pudding mix

2 tablespoon of honey

1 large grated pear

1/2 cup of coconut milk

3/4 cup of low-fat milk

INSTRUCTIONS

1. Bring the milk, vanilla pudding mix, coconut milk, pear and honey to a boil over medium heat, remove immediately from heat.

2. Stir in pudding gently with a wire whisk. Mix in shredded coconut, cooked rice and ginger. Allow the mixture to rest for 10

minutes for best favors, stirring once a bit. If desired top with berries. Served warm or chill before serving.

Nutrition information per servings:
Calories: 190 kcal
Carbohydrates: 3 g
Fat: 31g
Protein: 2g
Sodium: 244 mg

Blueberry Cherry Crisp

Prep time: 15 minutes
Cook time: 33-38 minutes
Servings: 8

INGREDIENTS

2 cups of frozen blueberries
4 cups of frozen cherries, thawed
1/8 tsp of sea salt
1/4 tsp of nutmeg
1 tsp of cinnamon
2 tbsp of honey
3 tbsp of butter
2 tbsp of coconut oil
1/2 cup of chopped macadamia nuts
1/3 cup of whole-wheat flour

INSTRUCTIONS

1. Heat up the oven to 375 degrees F.
2. Lightly grease a 9-x-9-inch baking glass dish with unsalted butter.

3. Mix together the flour, oatmeal and chopped macadamia nuts in a large bowl. Set one aside.

4. Combine together the cinnamon, butter, coconut oil, nutmeg, honey and sea salt in a small saucepan.

5. Place the mixture over low heat for about 3 minutes until the butter is melted. Stir butter/oil mixture and spread on top of the oatmeal mixture. Stir until you have a crumbly mixture.

6. Place the blueberries and the cherries in the prepared glass dish.

7. Place oatmeal mixture on top of the berries.

8. Place in the oven and bake until the topping has browned and crisp is bubbly, about 30 to 35 minutes. To Serve drizzle each crisp with a little of honey. 1-1/2 cups per serving.

Nutrition information per servings:
Calories: 252 kcal
Carbohydrates: 23 g
Fat: 16g
Protein: 4 g
Sodium: 38

Way Back Baked Apples with Filling

Prep time: 15 minutes

Cook time: 15 minutes

Servings: 4

INGREDIENTS

Dash of vanilla

Dash of nutmeg

1/4 tsp of cinnamon

1/3 cup of chopped pecans

3 tbsp of raisins

1 cup of apple juice

3/4 cup of tahini

4 ripe apples

3/4 cup of boiling water

INSTRUCTIONS

1. Heat up your oven to 375 degrees F. Lightly grease a 9-x-13-inch baking dish.

2. Remove each apple'score bottom to 1/2 inch with an apple corer or a paring knife; making wide holes of about 3/4 inch to 1 inch and remove seed with a spoon. Place the top side of the apples up in a shallow baking dish.

3. Mix half the apple juice and tahini together in a small bowl. Add the pecans, nutmeg, raisins, vanilla and cinnamon and mix together.

4. Pour the filling into each cored apple.

5. Pour hot water into the baking pan. Pour some of the reserved apple juice on top each apple.

6. Place in the oven and bake for 30 to 40 minutes until soft but not mushy.

7. Take the apples out of the oven and baste each apples multiple times with the remaining apple juices. Serve warm.

Nutrition information per servings:
Calories: 386 kcal
Carbohydrates: 34 g
Fat: 24g
Protein: 8 g
Sodium: 19 mg

Watermelon Apple And Cantaloupe Parfait

Prep time: 15 minutes
Cook time: 10 minutes
Servings: 4

INGREDIENTS

1 Cup of Watermelon seeded and chopped
1 Small Apple (Peeled, cored and chopped)
2 Cups of low-fat Granola (I used home-made)
16 Oz. of Low-fat Yogurt Whipped until smooth (unsweetened)
1 Cup of Sweet Cantaloupe Chopped

INSTRUCTIONS

1. Evenly divide the cantaloupe among 4 parfait glasses.
2. Add quarter cup of yogurt over cantaloupe in each glass. Add ¼ cup of granola.
3. Evenly divide the diced apple among the parfait glasses to make another layer.
Add quarter cup of yogurt over and quarter cup of granola in each glass.
4. Divide chopped watermelon evenly among 4 parfait glasses.
5. Top with the remaining 1/2 yogurt and 1/2 granola to garnish.

Nutrition information per servings:

Calories: 595 kcal
Carbohydrates: 100 g
Fat: 7g
Protein: 15 g
Sodium: 369 mg

Creamy Apples

Prep time: 15 minutes
Cook time: 20 minutes
Servings: 4

INGREDIENTS

140 grams of Fresh Raspberries
300 ml Greek Yogurt
2-3 tablespoon of water
1 teaspoon of ground cinnamon
1 tablespoon of Manuka Honey
450 grams of Apples Peeled, cored and chopped

INSTRUCTIONS

1. Place the chopped apples, cinnamon, honey and water in a saucepan and cook, stirring occasionally on low heat for 15 minutes or until the apples are tender and fluffy.
2. Remove apples from heat and beat until there are no lumps. Set aside.
3. In a large bowl, place the Greek yogurt, whip until smooth and then add in the apple mixture. Stir the raspberries into the yogurt-apple mixture but reserve a few for decoration.
4. Divide yogurt-apple among 4 dishes and place in the refrigerator to chill for up to hour. To serve garnish the reserved raspberries.

Nutrition information per servings:
Calories: 171 kcal
Carbohydrates: 26 g
Fat: 0.3gg
Protein: 8g
Sodium: 58 mg

Semi-frozen Strawberry With Balsamic Vinegar

Prep time: 90 minutes
Cook time: 10 minutes
Servings: 4

INGREDIENTS

4 Baby Strawberries
85 ml of Water
1 teaspoon of Manuka Honey
2 tablespoons of Balsamic Vinegar
150 gram of Ripe Strawberries cut in half

INSTRUCTIONS

1. Fast freeze the freezer at least two hours before placing this dessert.
2. Bring honey and water to a boil in a saucepan, stirring frequently. Reduce heat and simmer on low heat. Add in the strawberries and simmer for about 2 to 4 minutes. Set aside to cool.
3. Add the strawberries, syrup and balsamic vinegar in a food processor and process a few seconds until chunky.

4. Pour the mixture into a dish safe for the freezer and freeze for 60-90 minutes or until almost frozen. Stir once while the freezing.

5. Spoon the Semi frozen mixture into 4 individual dessert glasses. Decorate with baby strawberries. Don't forget to return the freezer to its formal setting.

Nutrition information per servings:
Calories: 66 kcal
Carbohydrates: 0.2 g
Fat: 0.3gg
Protein: 1g
Sodium: 2 mg

Baked Coated Tofu

Prep time: 5 minutes

Cook time: 20 minutes

Servings: 3

Low Sodium, Low Potassium, Low Phosphorus

INGREDIENTS

1 ½ cups of firm tofu (12 oz)

1 teaspoon of seasoning (paprika, garlic powder, curry, or other spice)

½ cup of cornflake crumbs

2 tablespoon of water

1 teaspoon of tamari sauce

INSTRUCTIONS

1. In a small mixing bowl, mix together water and tamari.

2. Pour cornflake crumbs in another bowl and mix in the seasoning.

3. Take the tofu and Dip into the tamari, then into the cornflake crumbs mixture.

4. Lightly wipe the baking sheet with vegetable oil and place the coated tofu onto the greased baking sheet.

5. Place in the oven and bake for 20 minutes at 350 degrees F, flip once to brown on each sides.

Nutrition information per servings:

Calories: 189 kcal

Carbohydrates: 9 g

Protein: 13g

Sodium: 148 mg

Pumpkin Pie vanilla Ice Cream

Prep time: 5 minutes

Cook time: 5 minutes

 Servings: 8

INGREDIENTS

1 (9 inches) baked pie shell

1 cup of whipped topping

1/4 tsp of nutmeg

1/2 tsp of cinnamon

1/2 tsp of ginger

Maple syrup

1 cup of canned pumpkin

2 cups of vanilla ice cream, softened

INSTRUCTIONS

1. Set the pie shell aside and mix all the ingredient in food processor until finely blended.

2. Transfer mixture into the pie shell, then place in the freezer to get firm.

Nutrition information per servings:

Calories: 152 kcal

Carbohydrates: 42 g

Protein: 3g

Sodium: 118 mg